How the NIH Can Help You Get Funded

HOW THE NIH CAN HELP YOU GET FUNDED: AN INSIDER'S GUIDE TO GRANT STRATEGY

MICHELLE L. KIENHOLZ
AND JEREMY M. BERG

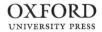

OXFORD
UNIVERSITY PRESS

Oxford University Press is a department of the University of Oxford.
It furthers the University's objective of excellence in research, scholarship,
and education by publishing worldwide.

Oxford   New York
Auckland   Cape Town   Dar es Salaam   Hong Kong   Karachi
Kuala Lumpur   Madrid   Melbourne   Mexico City   Nairobi
New Delhi   Shanghai   Taipei   Toronto

With offices in
Argentina   Austria   Brazil   Chile   Czech Republic   France   Greece
Guatemala   Hungary   Italy   Japan   Poland   Portugal   Singapore
South Korea   Switzerland   Thailand   Turkey   Ukraine   Vietnam

Oxford is a registered trademark of Oxford University Press
in the UK and certain other countries.

Published in the United States of America by
Oxford University Press
198 Madison Avenue, New York, NY 10016

Library of Congress Cataloging-in-Publication Data
Kienholz, Michelle L., author.
How the NIH can help you get funded : an insider's guide to grant strategy / Michelle L. Kienholz
and Jeremy M. Berg.
p. ; cm.
Includes index.
ISBN 978-0-19-998964-5 (alk. paper)
I. Berg, Jeremy M. (Jeremy Mark), 1958- author.   II. Title.
[DNLM: 1. National Institutes of Health (U.S.)   2. Biomedical Research—economics—United States.
3. Financing, Organized—United States.   4. Federal Government—United States.   5. Government
Agencies—United States.   6. Research Support, N.I.H., Extramural—United States. W 20.5]
R853.C55
610.72′4—dc23
2013025971

9 7 8 6 5
Printed in Canada
on acid-free paper

To all the researchers who have taught us so much by sharing their grant application experiences and allowing us to read the future in their proposals, and to the NIH staff members committed to shepherding this future into reality.

Contents

Foreword

THIS BOOK BY authors intimately familiar with the NIH is an outstanding guide to help scientists interact productively with the agency and develop competitive applications.

The mission of the NIH is to ensure that the best science by the most promising scientists is fairly reviewed and supported. This seemingly simple statement is overlaid on a complicated organization, with the Center for Scientific Review coordinating most of the reviews, and two dozen distinct Institutes and Centers, each with their own scientific priorities and culture, potentially funding applications.

I encountered this complexity, first as an applicant and grantee and then as a scientific advisor to the National Cancer Institute. However, I really came face-to-face with it when I became NIH Director. Indeed, my first major initiative was the development of the "NIH Roadmap for Medical Research". While the Roadmap included a number of important scientific initiatives and programs, the Roadmap was fundamentally designed to bring the institutes and centers together to develop and support great science that would advance the overall NIH goals. In other words, the Roadmap sought to harness the agency's complexity rather than be hampered by it.

Another of my other major initiatives involved streamlining the application and peer review process. The mantra of "Enhancing Peer Review" was to "fund the best science, by the best scientists, with the least amount of administrative burden". We reached out to many individuals and groups to hear their best ideas and then shaped these into a coherent plan. Our approach included adjusting the structure of grant applications, changing review formats, and carefully evaluating the impact of these changes to ensure that the "enhanced" processes were helping NIH achieve its goals as effectively as possible. This initiative also clarified the roles of the NIH review and program staff.

Unfortunately, these changes were superimposed on the aftermath the NIH budget doubling. As a consequence of the budget increases from 1998 to 2003, many investigators were joining the ranks of those competing for NIH funding over a period when the NIH budget did not even keep pace with inflation. The challenges of this decade-long trend have been exacerbated by the recent budget sequestration. In these days of highly constrained funding, transparent communication and information exchange between the NIH and the scientific community at large is essential.

This book will, I believe, be particularly helpful to young and new investigators, who are most at risk, but also to experienced investigators in communicating with NIH and navigating complex grant application processes to achieve ultimate success.

Kudos to the authors for a job well done!
Elias A. Zerhouni, MD
NIH Director, 2002–2008

Preface

AT SOME POINT, everyone interested in academic biomedical research is told he or she will need to "write a grant." Most have no idea what that means or where to start.

Although training programs are getting better about incorporating grant-writing courses or seminars, most investigators still have dozens of questions about the process, including many that they don't even know they have (or should have). There is so much more to developing an NIH grant proposal than just completing and submitting the application, though even that itself is daunting.

Both beginning and many established investigators do not know for whom to write or how much or what sort of detail to include. They do not realize they can and should take an active role in identifying potential review groups (before starting to write) and interacting with program staff at the NIH. They do not know how to make the connection, what they can ask, or when program staff will have answers. We have focused on helping investigators understand the NIH, how to work with staff, and how to use available data to their advantage in planning and preparing grant applications.

Furthermore, although it is not directly involved with the application process itself, the federal budget process routinely delays the NIH appropriation such that NIH staff often do not know whether or when an application might receive an award. We explain how these are tied together and also encourage those who are frustrated by low success rates to take our advice on how to advocate for more federal funding of biomedical research and to actively make their voice heard while Congress is deciding the NIH appropriation.

The importance of understanding the NIH as an institution and a federal agency brings up the other constituency we aim to help through the book: NIH extramural staff (program officers, scientific review officers, grants management specialists). By demystifying the process and helping investigators feel comfortable communicating with NIH personnel, we hope to make their future interactions more productive. By explaining where to find and how to use data already available from the NIH, we hope to make these future interactions more efficient as well. Our goal is to make the lives of program officers and other staff easier and allow everyone to focus on the science, which is more exciting for all involved.

Because the NIH is a single federal agency comprising 27 semiautonomous institutes and centers, finding a central source of information to address both the whole and the parts of most interest to an investigator is difficult. Over the years, we have each answered questions and provided guidance to investigators in person and through our respective blogs, and we were delighted when presented with the opportunity to combine and consolidate our insight and experience. We have identified common practices and highlighted differences among the Institutes and Centers in a broad sense, but we also remind you that policies and structure evolve continuously at the institution and the institute level, such that the book should serve as a guide rather than a definitive reference book. We wish you all the best success with your research and hope *How the NIH Can Help You Get Funded* helps you all do so.

Acknowledgments

WE ARE GRATEFUL to our editor at Oxford University Press, Chad Zimmerman, for his enthusiasm about our book and the NIH program officer who pointed him to the Medical Writing, Editing & Grantsmanship blog when he was seeking an author to prepare a book about NIH grant funding. We thank those Institute and Center Directors and other NIH staff who responded to our requests for information to compile in Chapter 2 and the Appendix and help convey the importance of understanding each Institute and Center individually. We have done our best to compile accurate and current information about the NIH and to integrate it correctly, but, no doubt, some errors will appear, for which we take full responsibility; we remind the reader also that Web sites may have been updated since the book went to print and funding opportunity links should be checked for any reissued announcements. We thank Jaideep Behari, Doris Rubio, Darren Sledjeski, Richard Steinman, Gary Thomas, and Michael Trakselis for reviewing our drafts and providing thoughtful feedback to ensure we were addressing the needs of our target audience. We thank David Whitcomb for allowing us to use his eRA Commons account to give new applicants a peek into what to expect. Most of all, we thank the hundreds of investigators who have asked questions and helped us understand what you need to know about applying for funding from the NIH.

Essential Steps for Securing NIH Grant Funding: A Quick Guide to Key Concepts

WE CREATED THIS overview page both to summarize the grant application planning and preparation process and to direct you to appropriate chapters in the book. In 15 easy steps, here is what you should do:

1. Come up with blockbuster, paradigm-shifting idea (BPSI) (this one is all you)
2. Identify the most appropriate funding opportunity announcement (FOA) based on research objectives, mechanism, and participating Institutes and Centers (ICs) (Chapters 2, 4, 6, and 7)
3. Check the current funding of science related to your BPSI (RePORTER, ICs) (Chapters 2, 4, and 6)
4. Contact the appropriate Program Officer (PO) at your target IC to discuss your BPSI and funding strategies (ICs, RePORTER, peers) (Chapters 2 and 10, Appendix)
5. Identify review groups who will be excited by your BPSI (Center for Scientific Review, RePORTER, PO, peers) (Chapters 3, 4, 6, and 10)
6. Organize and write your narrative for the majority of reviewers on your targeted study section (i.e., those who will not read the application or have expertise in your field) (Chapters 3 and 8)
7. Carefully craft the Specific Aims page to immediately hook and inspire your reviewers to enthusiastically present your application to the study section (Chapters 8 and 10)
8. Find colleagues and disinterested third-party readers to give feedback on what you are actually communicating through your narrative (might not be your BPSI) (Chapter 10)

9. Present an easy (text formatting) and enjoyable (writing style) narrative to read—be kind to your reviewers and do not create extra work for them (Chapter 9)

10. Write a cover letter that identifies your target IC, scientific review group, necessary reviewer expertise, and any conflicted reviewers (Chapter 8)

11. Work with the Scientific Review Officer to ensure that everything is in order for the review of your application (Chapters 3 and 11)

12. Wait to contact your PO until your summary statement is available (Chapters 10 and 11)

13. Understand that the federal budget status can dramatically affect when you may learn whether/when you will receive an award (Chapters 1, 5, and 12)

14. Communicate with your PO at all stages (presubmission, postsubmission, postaward) (Chapters 2, 10, 11, 12, 13, and 14)

15. Know what to do next, no matter the outcome of your application (Chapters 11, 12, 13, and 14)

Abbreviations

A0 = initial application

A1 = first amended application

AA = National Institute on Alcohol Abuse and Alcoholism (grant ID number abbreviation)

ACD = Advisory Committee to the Director

AG = National Institute on Aging (grant ID number abbreviation)

AI = National Institute of Allergy and Infectious Diseases (grant ID number abbreviation)

AOR = Authorized Organization Representative

AREA = Academic Research Enhancement Award (R15)

AR = National Institute of Arthritis and Musculoskeletal Diseases (grant ID number abbreviation)

AT = National Center for Complementary and Alternative Medicine (grant ID number abbreviation)

CA = National Cancer Center (grant ID number abbreviation)

CC = Clinical Center

CIT = Center for Information Technology

CR = Continuing Resolution

CSR = Center for Scientific Review

CTSA = Clinical and Translational Science Award

DA = National Institute on Drug Abuse (grant ID number abbreviation)

DC = National Institute on Deafness and Other Communication Disorders (grant ID number abbreviation)

DE = National Institute of Dental and Craniofacial Research (grant ID number abbreviation)

DK = National Institute of Diabetes and Digestive and Kidney Diseases (grant ID number abbreviation)

DPCPSI = Division of Program Coordination, Planning, and Strategic Initiatives

EB = National Institute of Biomedical Imaging and Bioengineering (grant ID number abbreviation)

eRA = Electronic Research Administration

ES = National Institute of Environmental Health Sciences (grant ID number abbreviation)

ESI = Early-Stage Investigator

EY = National Eye Institute (grant ID number abbreviation)

FASEB = Federation of American Societies of Experimental Biology

FIC = Fogarty International Center

FOA = Funding Opportunity Announcement

FY = Fiscal Year

GM = National Institute of General Medical Sciences (grant ID number abbreviation)

GMS = Grant Management Specialist

HD = National Institute of Child Health and Human Development (grant ID number abbreviation)

HG = National Human Genome Research Institute (grant ID number abbreviation)

HHS = Health and Human Services (US Department of)

HL = National Heart, Lung, and Blood Institute (grant ID number abbreviation)

IAM = Internet Assisted Meeting

IAR = Internet Assisted Review

IC = Institute or Center

IRG = Integrated Review Group

JIT = Just in Time

LOI = Letter of Intent

LM = National Library of Medicine (grant ID number abbreviation)

MD = National Institute on Minority Health and Health Disparities (grant ID number abbreviation)

MERIT = Method to Extend Research In Time (R37)

MH = National Institute of Mental Health (grant ID number abbreviation)

NCATS = National Center for Advancing Translational Sciences

NCCAM = National Center for Complementary and Alternative Medicine

NCI = National Cancer Institute

NEI = National Eye Institute

NHLBI = National Heart, Lung and Blood Institute

NHGRI = National Human Genome Research Institute

NIA = National Institute on Aging

NIAAA = National Institute on Alcohol Abuse and Alcoholism

NIAID = National Institute of Allergy and Infectious Diseases

NIAMS = National Institute of Arthritis and Musculoskeletal Diseases

NIBIB = National Institute of Biomedical Imaging and Bioengineering

NICHD = National Institute of Child Health and Human Development

NIDA = National Institute on Drug Abuse

NIDCD = National Institute on Deafness and Other Communication Disorders

NIDCR = National Institute of Dental and Craniofacial Research

NIDDK = National Institute of Diabetes and Digestive and Kidney Diseases

NIEHS = National Institute of Environmental Health Sciences

NIGMS = National Institute of General Medical Sciences

NIH = National Institutes of Health

NIMH = National Institute of Mental Health

NIMHD = National Institute on Minority Health and Health Disparities

NINDS = National Institute of Neurological Disorders and Stroke

NINR = National Institute of Nursing Research

NLM = National Library of Medicine

NoA = Notice of Award

NR = National Institute of Nursing Research (grant ID number abbreviation)

NRFC = Not Recommended for Further Consideration

NS = National Institute of Neurological Disorders and Stroke (grant ID number abbreviation)

OAR = Office of AIDS Research

OBSSR = Office of Behavioral and Social Sciences Research

OD = Office of the Director (of the NIH)

ODP = Office of Disease Prevention

OER = Office of Extramural Research

OMB = Office of Management and Budget (White House)

ORI = Office of Research Integrity

ORWH = Office of Research on Women's Health

OSC = Office of Strategic Coordination

PA = Program Announcement

PAR = Program Announcement Reviewed in an Institute (special receipt, referral, and/or review considerations)

PAS = Program Announcement with Set-Aside Funds

PD = Program Director

PI = Principal Investigator

PO = Program Officer

RCR = Responsible Conduct of Research

RePORT = Research Portfolio Online Reporting Tools

RFA = Request for Applications (grants, cooperative agreements)

RFP = Request for Proposals (contracts)

RPG = Research Project Grant (Roo, Ro1, Ro3, R15, R21, R34, R36, R37, R56, Po1, Uo1, U19, DPx, and other specialized mechanisms)

RPPR = Research Performance Progress Report

SBIR = Small Business Innovation Research

SEP = Special Emphasis Panel

SMRB = Scientific Management Review Board

SNAP = Streamlined Noncompeting Award Process

SRG = Scientific Review Group

SRO = Scientific Review Officer

STTR = Small Business Technology Transfer

TR = National Center for Advancing Translational Sciences (grant ID number abbreviation)

TW = Fogarty International Center (grant ID number abbreviation)

How the NIH Can Help You Get Funded

1

National Institutes of Health

THE NATIONAL INSTITUTES OF HEALTH (NIH) are just that—a collection of 27 Institutes and Centers (ICs) that collectively work to improve the health of the nation by each pursuing its own mission in its own way. Understanding how the entire agency (the NIH) and the individual ICs operate will help you plan your application strategy, seek assistance effectively, and understand when to expect funding decisions (and how they are made).

Although the roots of the NIH go back to the start of the nation, its start as a grant-making agency began in 1937 with the passage of the National Cancer Institute Act. The next year, the National Cancer Advisory Council approved the first applications for funding (fellowships), and the cornerstone of Building 1 on the NIH campus was laid. The history and development of the modern NIH is interesting, but we leave it to you to pursue as you wish (http://www.nih.gov/about/history.htm), as it is not critical for your grant-seeking strategy.

What is important to understand is how the NIH is managed legislatively. As part of the US Department of Health and Human Services, the NIH is in the executive branch of the federal government, which reports to the President. However, Congress both *authorizes* the NIH and *appropriates* funding.

Different committees handle these functions:

- The Senate Committee on Health, Education, Labor, and Pensions (http://help.senate.gov/) and the House Committee on Energy and Commerce (http://energycommerce.house.gov/subcommittees/health) are responsible for *authorization*.

- The Senate Subcommittee on Labor, Health and Human Services, Education, and Related Agencies (http://appropriations.senate.gov/sc-labor.cfm) and the House Subcommittee on Labor, Health and Human Services, Education, and Related Agencies (http://appropriations.house.gov/subcommittees/subcommittee/?IssueID=34777) are responsible for *appropriation* (i.e., the money).

Although the appropriation activity (explained in Chapter 5) is more important to you than the authorization, significant changes can be introduced when Congress reauthorizes the NIH (http://www.nih.gov/about/reauthorization/). For example, the National Institutes of Health Reform Act of 2006 established the Scientific Management Review Board to advise the NIH Director on the use of organizational authority (e.g., creating a new IC, abolishing an existing one, merging one or more, etc.) and to review the organization of the NIH at least once every 7 years.

Because Congress decides the fate of NIH funding each year, you are encouraged to contact your own elected delegation and the chairs of the Committees noted earlier to advocate for sustained, reliable increases in the NIH appropriation. This can be done as an individual constituent or through more coordinated activities run through scientific societies. The NIH budget was approximately doubled between 1998 and 2003, an effort spanning four Congresses, two Presidents, and two NIH Directors, but since then, the appropriation to the NIH has not kept pace with inflation and, in some years, has actually dropped. The NIH must be able to rely on a regular adjustment for inflation (if not more) each year so the ICs can count on funding levels and thus strategically plan multiple years ahead rather than be forced to be conservative in long-term commitments and scramble midway through each FY to estimate how many awards can be made. This will be explained further in Chapter 5.

At the top, the NIH Office of the Director sets cross-cutting policy but does not select applications for funding, except for some programs in the NIH Common Fund (originally developed as the NIH Roadmap (http://commonfund.nih.gov/index.aspx). As semiautonomous organizations, each with its own Congressionally authorized mission, the ICs determine which areas of science to emphasize through research initiatives, define funding plans and policies, determine how to allocate their appropriated funds among different mechanisms and activities, and decide which individual applications to fund. This is why Harold Varmus, who served as NIH Director from 1993 to 1999, expressed pleasure about being appointed Director of the National Cancer Institute in 2010, since he could finally be engaged in the actual selection of scientific projects to fund.

Three Centers at the NIH do not have funding authority: the Center for Scientific Review (CSR), the Clinical Center (CC), and the Center for Information Technology (CIT). Of these, we will only discuss CSR (Chapter 3), which is responsible for referring all applications to scientific review groups and managing the review process for 70% of applications submitted to the NIH. Chapter 2 discusses the culture and organization of the other 24 ICs.

You might also keep in mind that the process by which the NIH awards funding is mandated by Public Law (section 492 of the Public Health Service Act and federal regulations governing "Scientific Peer Review of Research Grant Applications and Research and Development Contract Projects" [42 CFR Part 52h, http://www.gpo.gov/fdsys/pkg/CFR-2007-title42-vol1/pdf/CFR-2007-title42-vol1-part52h.pdf]). This law sets up the two-stage review process and has buffered the NIH from Congressionally inserted earmarks relative to other agencies. As noted earlier, CSR manages most of the first-stage review of scientific merit, though the ICs also empanel study sections to review those applications specific to their mission (e.g., centers, career development, solicited applications). When your application is assigned for review, you will interact with NIH staff known as Scientific Review Officers (SROs), who select experts to review assigned applications, manage study section meetings, and prepare summary statements (more on this in Chapter 3).

Approximately 80% of the NIH budget ($31 billion in fiscal year 2012) funds extramural research through grants and contracts, predominantly in the United States, with small amounts going to researchers in other countries. Within the NIH, approximately 11% goes toward intramural research conducted by the ICs, approximately 5% goes to the support of agency staff and administration, and approximately 2.5% supports formal training programs. Each IC has its own management style (Chapter 2), but they all seek to maximize the amount of funding available to support extramural research. You will interact with extramural staff known as Program Officers (POs) and, if you receive an award, Grants Management Specialists (GMSs). Again, each IC and each PO has individual preferences for how and when you interact, but the take-home point is that you as an applicant are encouraged to contact NIH staff at each stage of the application, review, and award process. You should not be shy about asking questions and should not assume that inter-acting with institute personnel is inappropriate. We will explain the etiquette for such interactions and what questions or behavior might be out of bounds in Chapter 10.

NIH-wide policy related to the solicitation, funding, and management of extramural research is developed in response to regulations set by the US Department of Health and Human Services, by the NIH authorization act (as noted earlier, updated periodically by Congress), and based on feedback from the extramural research community. The Office of Extramural Research (Chapter 4), which is part of the Office of the Director, is responsible for formulating and publishing new NIH-wide policy and coordinating its implementation across the ICs.

Office of the Director

Although you are not likely to interact with the Director of the NIH, you might find useful resources and contacts in several offices administra-tively housed within the Division of Program Coordination, Planning, and Strategic Initiatives (DPCPSI) (http://dpcpsi.nih.gov) of the Office of the Director (OD). Some of these offices allocate extramural research funding and have program staff whom you may wish to contact when planning your research and preparing an application.

- *Office of AIDS Research* (OAR, http://www.oar.nih.gov)—OAR coordinates the scientific, budgetary, legislative, and policy elements of NIH AIDS research (both extra- and intramural). OAR allocates all appropriated AIDS research funds to the ICs according to the Trans-NIH Plan for HIV-Related Research. OAR also reviews grants and contracts supported by AIDS-designated funds, which are allocated to ICs based not on a formula, but on the priorities of the Plan, scientific opportunities, and the capacity of individual ICs to support the most meritorious science.
- *Office of Behavioral and Social Sciences Research* (OBSSR, http://obssr. od.nih.gov/index.aspx)—OBSSR focuses on behavioral, psychological, socioeconomic, sociodemographic, and cultural research. Although OBSSR does not have grant-making authority, it does develop and issue funding opportunity announcements (FOAs) for which it transfers

funds to the participating ICs, which in turn administer the awarded applications. OBSSR also facilitates the NIH Basic Behavioral and Social Science Opportunity Network (OppNet, http://oppnet.nih.gov), a trans-NIH initiative that "prioritizes activities and initiatives that focus on basic mechanisms of behavior and social processes."

- *Office of Disease Prevention* (ODP, http://prevention.nih.gov/default. aspx)—ODP coordinates research activities related to disease prevention, dietary supplements, and medical applications of research but does not allocate funding in these areas. ODP also manages the NIH Consensus Development Program (http://prevention.nih.gov/cdp/default.aspx).
- *Office of Research on Women's Health* (ORWH, http://orwh.od.nih. gov)—ORWH coordinates and cofunds women's health and sex differences research. Working in partnership with the ICs, ORWH also supports women engaged in NIH research, especially minority women, and the career development of scientists focused on women's health research.
- *Office of Strategic Coordination* (OSC, https://commonfund.nih.gov)— OSC manages the NIH Common Fund programs, such as the various NIH Director awards (Pioneer, New Innovator, Early Independence, Transformative Research), and many special initiatives. The Common Fund supports NIH-wide initiatives addressing major topics and technologies that no single institute or center could manage alone. Congress directly appropriates Common Fund levels and may include recommendations for research priorities (but does not assign specific dollar amounts to any topic area).

In addition, a variety of advisory groups provide guidance to the NIH Director:

- *Scientific Management Review Board* (http://smrb.od.nih.gov), which advises the HHS and NIH officials on the use of organizational authorities regarding NIH ICs and the Office of the Director
- *Advisory Committee to the Director* (http://acd.od.nih.gov), which assists with making major plans and policies, particularly with regard to the allocation of NIH funds and resources
- *Council of Councils* (http://dpcpsi.nih.gov/council/), which advises the Director on the policies and activities of DPCPSI and serves as an external advisory panel during the "concept clearance" stage of the NIH Common Fund review process

- *Council of Public Representatives* (http://www.nih.gov/about/copr/index.htm), which advises the Director on issues related to outreach and public participation in NIH activities

How an Application Becomes a Grant

Although the slang usage is to say you are "writing a grant," you are, of course, working on an application to receive a research grant—versus a loan or a contract. From the NIH, a grant is an assistance mechanism that provides money, resources, or both to the awardee to carry out an approved project. The administering IC has little or no programmatic involvement in the activities being carried out with the support of a grant, thus affording the principal investigator significant freedom in carrying out the project. There is no expectation of a specified service or end product for use by the IC.

A cooperative agreement (U mechanism) is used to provide this financial support when there will be substantial scientific or programmatic involvement by IC or other federal personnel with the awarded project.

A contract is used by the NIH to acquire goods or services that meet a specific need, such as operating a service facility, analyzing chemical compounds, or developing an animal model. Unlike grant and cooperative agreement funding announcements, contract opportunities are released as requests for proposals (RFPs) as Notices in the NIH Guide to Grants and Contracts (http://grants1.nih.gov/grants/guide/search_results.htm?year=active&scope=not).

In preparing your application, you are laying out your best scientific ideas and methods to achieve your objectives, your peers are evaluating the likelihood that your work will have a significant and lasting impact on the field and public health, and the IC is deciding whether your project best satisfies the current priorities within their strategic plan. If successful, you will be awarded a grant to conduct research as you see fit based on your findings. If your first application (designated as A0) is not successful, you only have one more opportunity to submit the research in an amended application (designated as A1). Chapter 13 reviews your options if your application will not be funded, including revising your A0 application for submission as an A1.

We will review the budget process (Chapter 5) and suggest strategies for preparing the application (Chapters 8 and 9) and interacting with NIH staff (Chapters 2 and 10), but here we present an overview of the timing of major events in the NIH-funded biomedical research enterprise.

The first column of Table 1.1 illustrates how Congressional action on the federal budget dictates the timing of NIH funding activities. Sadly, Congress has not passed appropriation bills in time for the new fiscal year (FY), which begins on October 1, in well over a decade, which means the federal government operates under a continuing resolution (CR) until one or more appropriation bills are passed by Congress and signed into law by the President; often Congress ends up passing one omnibus budget bill rather than individual appropriations bills for specific executive agencies. As detailed in Chapter 5, because the ICs do not know how much money they will have to spend during the FY, they must be fiscally conservative at the outset. At the start of the FY, the NIH often cuts all noncompeting renewal (that is, applications that were originally funded in prior FYs) budgets up to 10%, and ICs make awards to only the most competitive and most high-priority applications. Because they cannot be sure their appropriation will go up in subsequent FYs, the ICs must also be conservative in making awards for the long term, to ensure they can meet the obligations of noncompeting renewals in future years while also having money to make new awards.

The second column illustrates how far in advance ICs must plan special initiatives to be funded by monies set aside in a future FY appropriation (which can be identified as "cleared concepts" before the funding announcements are issued) as well as the timing of payline and funding decisions.

The third column estimates the timing and time requirements of the application process from the perspective of a principal investigator (PI) in terms of submitting applications, both to standard and Request for Application (RFA) receipt dates, including interactions with the PO. As a PI, you will, of course, be continuously conducting the research at the heart of the application, preparing and submitting manuscripts, meeting with collaborators to plan experiments, and other routine activities not explicitly indicated in the table. The major steps of preparing for and preparing your application include the following:

- Developing the idea—confirm it is of interest to one or more ICs, confirm similar research is not already being funded (check with PO [Chapter 2] and use RePORTER [Chapter 4])
- Identifying an appropriate mechanism (Chapter 7) and FOA for this idea (use OER and RePORTER; Chapter 4)
- Identifying appropriate reviewers for this idea—if none of the CSR SRGs will get excited about your science, you will be less likely to be scored well (use CSR [Chapter 3] and RePORTER [Chapter 4])

Table 1.1 The Timeline According to Which Applications Become Grants

2012   **FY12**

	Congress	ICs	PI	Standard FOAs
Jan	FY12 budget enacted		Preliminary data	
Feb	President's FY13 budget		R01 research project developed—meet PO	FY13 Cycle 1 receipt
Mar	Congressional committee meetings	Planning meetings for FY14 and FY15 budget	R01 application preparation	
Apr				
May				FY13 Cycle 2 receipt
June			Submit R01 A0 for Cycle 2, FY13	FY13 Cycle 1 review
July				
Aug	House-Senate-Conference			
Sept				
Oct	FY13 CR (no appropriation bills passed)	Interim FY13 paylines until appropriation passed—FY14 budget request	R01 A0 reviewed, score 45	FY13 Cycle 2 review
Nov			Summary statement reviewed with PO, revisions planned, additional experiments	FY13 Cycle 3 receipt
Dec			FY13 Cycle 1 award	

	2013						
FY13	Jan	FY13 CR	Conservative funding decisions for Cycle 1, FY13	Publication	FY13 Cycle 1 award		FY13 Cycle 3 review
	Feb			Revise R01			
	Mar	FY13 sequestration		Submit R01 A1 for Cycle 1, FY14			
	Apr	FY13 final appropriation passed/signed, FY14 budget introduced				FY13 Cycle 2 award	
	May		Final paylines/paylists when budget known and all three cycles reviewed				
	June			R01 A1 reviewed, score 28			
	July		Final awards for applications from all three cycles	Summary statement reviewed with PO, PO presents application at paylist meeting, not selected for funding			FY13 Cycle 3 award
	Aug						
	Sept						
	Oct	FY14 CR, if no appropriation bills passed/signed into law		PO suggests cleared concept for FY15 RFA			
	Nov		Prepare and issue RFA	Preliminary data specific to RFA			
	Dec						

(*continued*)

Table 1.1 (Continued)

		Congress	ICs	PI	Standard FOAs
FY14	Jan	FY14 CR may last into next calendar		Prepare RFA R01	
	Feb				
	Mar	year	RFA receipt	Submit revised R01 to	
	Apr	FY14 appropriation or omnibus bill		FY15 RFA	
	May				
	June	passed, signed into law	RFA review	RFA R01 reviewed, score 18	
	July			Summary statement reviewed with PO	
	Aug			PO advocates at paylist meeting	
	Sept		Council meeting	Application approved for funding	
FY15	Oct	FY15 CR, if no appropriation			
	Nov				
	Dec			Award issued	
	Jan				
	Feb				

CR, continuing resolution; FOA, funding opportunity announcement; FY, fiscal year; ICs, Institutes and Centers; PI, principal investigator; PO, program officer; RFA, request for application.

- Considering the review criteria (especially Approach, Significance, and Innovation) in laying out your ideas and drafting the narrative portions (Chapter 8)
- Preparing a clear, concise, compelling, easily followed narrative (Chapters 8 and 9)
- Seeking feedback from others (Chapter 10)

The final column (further broken into columns for each of the three cycles) lays out the timing of receipt, review, and award of applications submitted to standard funding cycles for FY13.

As will be discussed in subsequent chapters, your PO will not know whether your score and percentile will be "within the payline" or considered for select pay until Council meets—and until the IC knows its final appropriation (more on what all these terms mean in Chapters 3 and 11). Thus, conversations with your PO should wait until you have your summary statement in hand and you can discuss revising the application or reworking the application for a different mechanism, depending on your review outcome and submission status (A0 vs. A1).

2

Institutes and Centers

AS WE DISCUSSED in Chapter 1, the NIH is not a monolith but rather a collection of semiautonomous Institutes and Centers (ICs), each with its own culture and policies. Here we introduce you to the IC-specific personnel who will be most involved with your application (Program Officers and the Advisory Council) and summarize the funding trends and policies of the 24 ICs with funding authority, including their general approach to making funding decisions. Where available, we include funding trend data showing the number of applications scored and funded at each percentile. We separately provide in the Appendix a common dataset for each IC that will help you identify the right people and resources to guide your research and application development efforts.

Program Officers

As we will discuss in detail in Chapter 10 and throughout the book, your best friend in planning and submitting an application will be a Program Officer (PO). POs (also known as Program Officials) are IC extramural staff who administer scientific programs, oversee grant portfolios, set priorities, and act as an advocate for a scientific area—and for researchers in that area. They work closely with Scientific Review Officers (SROs), both at the Center for Scientific Review (CSR, Chapter 3) and within the IC, and Grant Management Specialists (GMSs) and assist investigators before and after the submission and review of the application and after an award is issued, for those principal investigators (PIs) whose applications are funded.

Although many investigators do not realize they can contact a PO, in fact, not only is such interaction allowed, it is strongly encouraged. Since POs were often previously investigators themselves, they remain deeply engaged with the research in their portfolio and come to look at these PIs as "their investigators." This theme will come up again in the next chapter, where your goal in communicating with the assigned reviewers on your study section is to have them come to think of you as one of "their investigators." You should contact program staff throughout the application process, starting in the planning stages of your application (Chapter 10 gives tips on finding and working with POs).

In an ideal world, your research will be of interest to more than one IC, so you can tap into different pots of money, in which case you will want to make connections with POs at each IC that might consider funding your work. We include in the Appendix links to lists of program staff at each IC: most are listed by scientific area of interest and would be contacted if you are working on a research project grant (RPG), but there are also staff assigned specifically to help with training, career development, and small business applications. Please review Chapter 10 for details on what you can and should discuss with your PO (and when) and etiquette tips for ensuring productive interactions.

Getting back to the ICs more broadly, you should keep in mind that they are all organized and managed individually and have widely varying cultures in terms of how their extramural research program is operated. Some run a tight ship, some are more relaxed. Of course, you apply to ICs based on scientific foci, not management style, but you want to keep in mind that the experience of your colleague who works with Institute X might not apply to your interactions at Institute Y. Interestingly, personnel at the ICs themselves, being inwardly focused, often do not realize how different they can be from one another.

Advisory Councils

Each IC also has its own Advisory Council or Board to conduct the second level of application review—though it is the IC Director, with guidance from senior staff, not Council, who makes the final award decisions. Councils are composed of scientists from the extramural research community and public representatives (http://ofacp.od.nih.gov/committees/index.asp). Members are selected by the Department of Health and Human Services, usually based on input from the ICs and the NIH Office of the Director. Most Councils meet (http://citfm.cit.nih.gov/ofacp/meetings.php) three times a year, in parallel with the standard application cycles; those for the National

Cancer Institute (NCI) and the National Institute of Heart, Lung and Blood Institute (NHLBI) meet four times a year (per early NIH legislation).

Chapter 11 reviews what happens at Advisory Council meetings and what it means for your application, and you can read the operations procedures for each IC on their Council Website (see Appendix). Briefly, about 2 months prior to the next scheduled meeting, Council members receive access to the summary statements and applications under consideration for funding (Council members cannot see these materials for applications from their own institution). Council considers whether the proposed research fits with the IC's mission rather than its scientific merit as well as the adequacy of the review, and members are asked to concur with the review. Some of the concurrence voting occurs electronically prior to the meeting, particularly for applications that scored very well. Exceptions include applications with any foreign involvement, from PIs receiving $1 million or more in NIH support, or with any unresolved concerns related to human subjects or vertebrate animal protection, biohazards, recruitment, or data monitoring, though a Council member can request that any application be discussed at the meeting. Council members also consider appeals from PIs who have a specific concern, such as evidence of bias in their study section review (http://grants.nih.gov/grants/guide/notice-files/not-od-11-064.html), as well as MERIT awards and extensions. As just noted, they review administrative concerns about applications being considered as well as proposals from foreign applicants.

Council also hears presentations about the research conducted at (intramural) and funded by (extramural) the IC and reviews "concepts" for future initiatives that may be awarded as grants, contracts, or cooperative agreements. These are called "cleared concepts" and once approved ("cleared") by Council, they will likely show up within the next several months as a Request for Applications (RFA) or Program Announcement Reviewed in an Institute (PAR) or as a Notice (for contracts) in the NIH Guide. If you monitor concepts as they are cleared, you can get a head start on preparing applications for these opportunities, which generally have short time frames. Your PO will also know more about them and be able to help with your advance planning.

The ICs also have Boards of Scientific Counselors, who review the intramural research programs, and various program advisory committees to provide guidance on developing extramural research initiatives. You would do well to familiarize yourself with all the advisory committees, their missions, and their reports at the IC(s) from which you seek funding.

Institutes and Centers Data

Here we present funding data for all the Institutes followed by the Centers (listed alphabetically by name, not abbreviation) as well as useful resources in developing your grant application and overall strategy. You will find the additional resources listed for the National Institute of Allergy and Infectious Diseases (http://www.niaid.nih.gov/researchfunding/grant/pages/aag.aspx) extremely helpful no matter where you seek funding at the NIH.

You should check the mission and priorities of ICs you are considering targeting and take note of the size of their appropriation; smaller ICs have less money but also generally less competition, so do not hesitate to check with POs about the suitability of your research for their portfolio.

Some of the data presented here may raise points of discussion with your PO (e.g., National Center for Complementary and Alternative Medicine, NCCAM, trend of not funding renewal Ro1s). Each IC also has its own new and early-stage investigator (ESI) policy (see Chapter 4 for NIH policy), which often influences funding decisions.

The Appendix adds information to help you navigate each IC Web site more efficiently and make contact with program staff. Please remember that IC Web sites are continually updated (in particular, more will likely add funding trend data) and that you may need to search for information that has moved. You can also check the Writedit blog (http:writedit.wordpress. com) for current links to funding data as well as paylines and other resources (members of the extramural community post their questions and experiences at http://writedit.wordpress.com/nih-paylines-resources).

National Cancer Institute (NCI)

> Web site: http://cancer.gov
> FY12 appropriation: $5.07B (FY13: $4.8B) (1st/24, established 1937)
> Mission: http://www.cancer.gov/aboutnci/overview/mission
> Funding decisions: http://deainfo.nci.nih.gov/grantspolicies/
>   FinalFundLtr.pdf

Scores and percentiles assigned through scientific peer review set the threshold for funding decisions, which are made by NCI Scientific Program Leaders (SPLs) following discussions with program staff. The SPLs give special consideration to applications that fill a significant gap in the cancer research portfolio or propose an especially novel or promising scientific approach.

Those within the "hard" payline (see for the current fiscal year funding strategy for latest threshold) will be funded, with few exceptions.

Funding Trends

- Does not participate in the R21 or R03 parent announcements but does offer an omnibus program announcement for the R21 mechanism (PAR-12-145) (R03 omnibus PAR-12-144 expired early)
- FY12 overall success rate (all mechanisms): 13.6%
- FY12 RPG success rate: 12.3% (new), 30.6% (renewal), 12.0% (supplement)
- FY12 R01 success rate: 12.5% (new), 29.4% (renewal), 11.8% (supplement)
- https://gsspubssl.nci.nih.gov/roller/ncidea/entry/2012_funding_patterns
- For R01 funding trend, see Figure 2.1.

Additional Resources

- Budget analysis tool: http://budgettool.cancer.gov

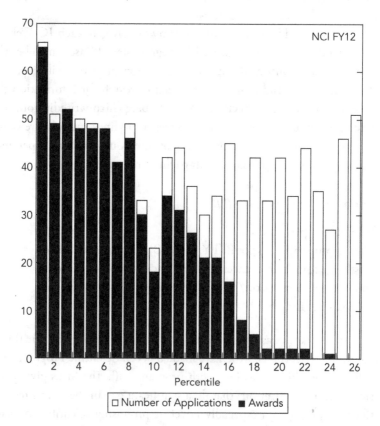

FIGURE 2.1 National Cancer Institute: number of R01 applications versus awards, FY2012.

- Fact book: http://obf.cancer.gov/financial/factbook.htm (detailed breakdown of budget expenditures, funding trends, extramural programs, organization charts)
- Funded research portfolio: http://fundedresearch.cancer.gov/

National Eye Institute (NEI)

Web site: http://www.nei.nih.gov
FY12 appropriation: $702M (FY13: $662M) (12th/24, established 1968)
Mission: http://www.nei.nih.gov/about/mission.asp
Funding decisions: http://nei.nih.gov/funding/ (scroll to link for Fiscal Operations Plan for current FY)

As part of the NEI approach to support new investigators on R01-equivalent grant awards at a success rate equal to that of established investigators, aproximately 60% of these new investigators will be ESI. The NEI also maintains the portfolio-average length of grants at 4 years by funding approximately equal numbers of 3-, 4-, and 5-year awards, which will help ensure that equivalent numbers of continuing applications will compete for funds in future years.

Funding Trends
- Does not participate in the R03 parent announcement
- FY12 overall success rate (all mechanisms): 29.8%
- FY12 RPG success rate: 22.9% (new), 48.3% (renewal), 33.3% (supplement)
- FY12 R01 success rate: 26.7% (new), 48.3% (renewal), 33.3% (supplement)

Additional Resources
Application guidelines: http://nei.nih.gov/funding/special.asp

National Heart, Lung and Blood Institute (NHLBI)

Web site: http://www.nhlbi.nih.gov/
FY12 appropriation: $3.07B (FY13: $2.9B) (3rd/24, established 1948)
Mission: http://www.nhlbi.nih.gov/about/org/mission.htm
Funding decisions: http://www.nhlbi.nih.gov/funding/genfund.htm

Much of the award strategizing at the NHLBI occurs prior to review (thus heightening the importance of communicating with your PO in advance).

The NHLBI is increasingly working with the investigator community to identify the most important questions, what kind of investments actually pay off, and opening up closed research communities where they believe research would have more impact if more players were in the game. The NHLBI believes all the clinical research should have some return on investment, unlike basic science research, which should be designed to explore, not build, and in which return decades later is not uncommon.

Funding Trends

- Does not participate in the R03 or R21 parent announcements
- FY12 overall success rate (all mechanisms): 14.7%
- FY12 RPG success rate: 13.3% (new), 26.3% (renewal), 25.0% (supplement)
- FY12 R01 success rate: 13.0% (new), 25.4% (renewal), 33.3% (supplement)

Additional Resources

Fact book: http://www.nhlbi.nih.gov/about/factpdf.htm or
http://www.nhlbi.nih.gov/about/factbook/toc.htm

National Human Genome Research Institute (NHGRI)

Web site: http://www.genome.gov
FY12 appropriation: $513M (FY13: $483M) (15th/24, established 1989)
Mission: http://www.genome.gov/10001022
Funding decisions:
http://www.genome.gov/ResearchFunding/(scroll down to PDF for
current FY Funding Policy)

The NHGRI does not have a payline nor does it have a set aside for "select pay." However, program staff and Council may designate applications as having high programmatic relevance in cases such as filling a gap in a research area, adding value to the research portfolio, nurturing emerging areas of science, encouraging the career development of individuals who have expertise necessary to further the research mission of the NHGRI, and so on. In very rare cases, program staff and Council may designate competitively scored applications as having low programmatic relevance. In both cases, these recommendations resulting from the Council discussions are taken into account when funding decisions are made.

Following each Council round, a list of eligible applications is generated that includes applications from the current Council and the two previous Councils. Applications from all three science divisions are merged in one document but are separated out according to activity codes so that similar research applications are considered together. Within each section, applications are listed in descending order of impact scores.

All POs are expected to attend the paylist meetings, at which time each PO will briefly describe, for each assigned application, the proposed research, summarize the initial reviewers' comments, and indicate whether and how the application is responsive to the Strategic Plan (http://www.genome.gov/27543215). Additional factors taken into consideration include whether the applicant is a new or early stage investigator or the first renewal application; Council's designation of applications for high or low programmatic relevance and its recommendations for applications subjected to Special Council Review; a PI's other sources of funding; and whether this is a revised application or the only source of funding for a PI's research. The PO also recommends a budget and project duration.

In general, most applications are awarded for 3 years, unless they are programs that would benefit from stability, such as training grants, career development awards, resource grants, or a special program commitment, such as Centers of Excellence in Genomic Science and Centers of Excellence in Ethical, Legal, and Social Implications (ELSI) Research. Before an application is placed on the paylist, all staff must concur with the PO's recommendation. Since there are three Councils per year, there are at least three paylist meetings. In general, funding is very conservative during the first two paylist meetings, with final decisions made about how much further to go down the eligible list applications (from all three cycles) made at the last paylist meeting. The NHGRI Director makes the final funding decisions based on recommendations from the POs.

By law, the ELSI program must account for 5% of the NHGRI extramural program budget. The process described earlier is also used to make funding decisions on ELSI applications. Individual fellowships are handled differently. Since they do not go to Council, the second level of review is conducted by an ad hoc group of POs, based on the science proposed, with these recommendations given to the NHGRI Director.

Funding Trends

- FY12 overall success rate (all mechanisms): 23.9%
- FY12 RPG success rate: 23.1% (new), 38.1% (renewal), 0% (supplement)
- FY12 R01 success rate: 23.2% (new), 35.0% (renewal), 0% (supplement)

Additional Resources
Funded research: http://www.genome.gov/10001799

National Institute on Aging (NIA)

Web site: http://www.nia.nih.gov
FY12 appropriation: $1.1B (FY13: $1.0B) (9th/24, established 1974)
Mission: http://www.nia.nih.gov/about/mission
Funding decisions: http://www.nia.nih.gov/research/dea/
nia-specific-policies

The NIA funds most research in order of percentile obtained in review, for applications reviewed by CSR. The Institute has discontinued use of percentiles for RPG applications that are reviewed by NIA study sections. These applications are considered separately from other RPG applications and have a separate funding line based upon priority/impact score and available funds. The Institute will allocate to this line no more than the average share of the funds expended on these kinds of competing awards for the preceding 2 years. Together, these funding pools account for 85% to 90% of NIA's extramural research funding.

The NIA also funds research addressing Institute priorities established through consultation with research and public communities, an internal planning process, and discussion with the National Advisory Council on Aging. About 3.4% of the Institute's annual RPG budget goes to three high-priority public health projects that serve as infrastructure for investigator-initiated and other designated priority research: the Alzheimer's Disease Neuroimaging Initiative, the Alzheimer's Disease Cooperative Study, and the Health and Retirement Study. These projects also receive support from other organizations at NIH, other agencies of the federal government, and from the private sector. In addition, the NIA issues RFAs each year in targeted areas related to its priorities. A smaller pool of discretionary funds is also allocated to support applications that score beyond the regular paylines but are responsive to NIA priorities. The RFA and discretionary pools together account for 10% to 15% of NIA's research funding.

The NIA has a tougher payline for "large" applications requesting more than $500,000 in direct costs in any of the requested budget years and has a cap for total dollars that the Institute accepts in a single year across all large applications. The NIA excludes R03 and R21 awards from administrative cuts.

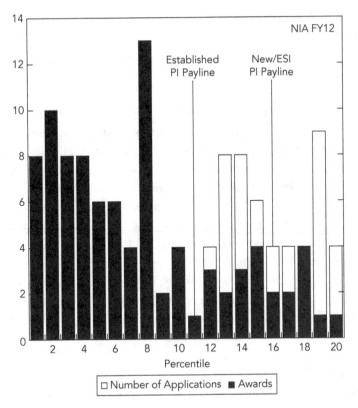

FIGURE 2.2 National Institute on Aging: number of R01 applications versus awards, FY2012.

Funding Trends

- FY12 overall success rate (all mechanisms): 15.5%
- FY12 RPG success rate: 13.5% (new), 34.6% (renewal), 25.0% (supplement)
- FY12 R01 success rate: 12.9% (new), 35.4% (renewal), 20.0% (supplement)
- For R01 funding trend, see Figure 2.2.

Additional Resources

Scientific resources: http://www.nia.nih.gov/research/scientific-resources
Inside NIA: a blog for researchers: http://www.nia.nih.gov/research/blog

National Institute of Alcohol Abuse and Alcoholism (NIAAA)

Web site: http://www.niaaa.nih.gov
FY12 appropriation: $459M (FY13: $433M)(16th/24, established)

Mission: http://www.niaaa.nih.gov/about-niaaa
Funding decisions:
http://www.niaaa.nih.gov/grant-funding/management-reporting/
    funding-procedures

Funding decisions are made during paylist meetings, where applications are discussed and prioritized, beginning with the top-scoring applications. After the discussion of the funding consideration for top-scoring applications, the paylist meeting staff review the applications up to about a specific percentile rank (R01) and equivalent priority score (other mechanisms), which are determined by the Budget Office. The NIAAA is committed to ensure that the overall success rate for new investigators approximates that for established investigators.

The critical factor for the final funding decisions is the budget availability. POs negotiate a lower funding level for applications that score well but have high costs. Applications below the payline may be recommended by program staff for "select pay" based on high program priority, cost, and new investigator status. The select paylist is reviewed by the Director and senior staff, with all final decisions made by the Director.

Funding Trends

- http://www.niaaa.nih.gov/grant-funding/management-reporting/
  funding-curves
- FY12 overall success rate (all mechanisms): 18.4%
- FY12 RPG success rate: 16.4% (new), 39.5% (renewal), 25.0% (supplement)
- FY12 R01 success rate: 14.4% (new), 22.8% (renewal), 50.0% (supplement)

Additional Resources

- Guidelines and resources: http://www.niaaa.nih.gov/research/
  guidelines-and-resources

National Institute of Allergy and Infectious Diseases (NIAID)

Web site: http://www.niaid.nih.gov
FY12 appropriation: $4.5B (FY13: $4.2B) (2nd/24, established 1955)
Mission: http://www.niaid.nih.gov/about/whoweare/Pages/default.aspx
Funding decisions: http://www.niaid.nih.gov/researchfunding/paybud/
    Pages/default.aspx
http://www.niaid.nih.gov/researchfunding/grant/strategy/
    Pages/7fundingdec.aspx

The NIAID funds all applications that rank within the payline, reflecting their scientific merit as judged by their peer reviewers. POs nominate a small number of programmatically important R01 applications that score above the payline; if Council approves, such applications may receive 4 years of funding.

Funding Trends
- FY12 overall success rate (all mechanisms): 23.2%
- FY12 RPG success rate: 20.7% (new), 44.1% (renewal), 46.7% (supplement)
- FY12 R01 success rate: 15.9% (new), 34.3% (renewal), 33.3% (supplement)
- For R01 funding trend, see Figure 2.3.

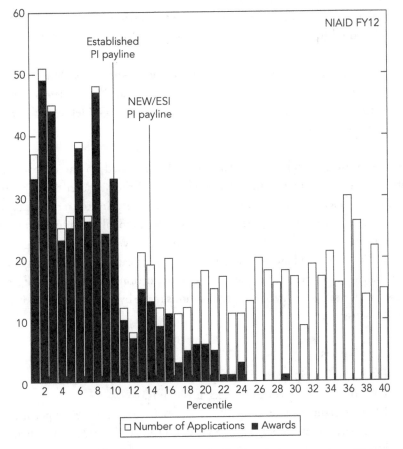

FIGURE 2.3 National Institute of Allergy and Infectious Diseases: number of R01 applications versus awards, FY2012.

Additional Resources

- Grant tutorials and tools: http://www.niaid.nih.gov/researchfunding/grant/pages/aag.aspx
- Sample applications and summary statements: http://www.niaid.nih.gov/researchfunding/grant/Pages/appsamples.aspx
- NIAID funding newsletter: http://www.niaid.nih.gov/researchfunding/newsletter/Pages/default.aspx
- Resources for researchers: http://www.niaid.nih.gov/labsandresources/resources/Pages/default.aspx

National Institute of Arthritis and Musculoskeletal and Skin Diseases (NIAMS)

Web site: http://www.niams.nih.gov/
FY12 appropriation: $535M (FY13: $505M) (14th/24, established)
Mission: http://www.niams.nih.gov/About_Us/Mission_and_Purpose/mission.asp
Funding decisions: http://www.niams.nih.gov/About_Us/Budget/funding_plan_fy2013.asp (click on most recent FY in the left column)
http://www.niams.nih.gov/Funding/Policies_and_Guidelines/funding_decisions.asp

The decision to fund a particular application is based on the outcome of its scientific merit review and on the relevance of the proposed work to the Institute's scientific and health priorities. Institute priorities reflect public health needs, scientific opportunities, and congressional and administration mandates, among other factors. At any point in a given fiscal year, budgetary projections are based on awarding funds to all applications with rankings better than a certain percentile (payline); a small portion of each year's budget is reserved for select pay awards, with decisions made by the Director following staff discussion.

Funding Trends

- Does not participate in the R03 parent announcement
- FY12 overall success rate (all mechanisms): 15.6%
- FY12 RPG success rate: 13.6% (new), 34.0% (renewal), 28.6% (supplement)
- FY12 R01 success rate: 12.8% (new), 32.1% (renewal), 33.3% (supplement)
- http://www.niams.nih.gov/About_Us/Budget/pattern_fy2012.asp
- For R01 funding trend, see Figure 2.4.

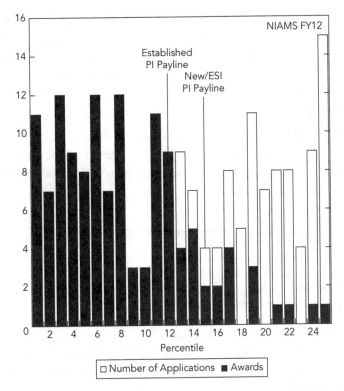

FIGURE 2.4 National Institute of Arthritis and Musculoskeletal and Skin Diseases: number of R01 applications versus awards, FY2012.

Additional Resources

- Research and training mechanisms: http://www.niams.nih.gov/ Funding/Funding_Opportunities/activity_codes.asp
- Funded research: http://www.niams.nih.gov/Funding/Funded_ Research/default.asp

National Institute of Biomedical Imaging and Bioengineering (NIBIB)

Web site: http://www.nibib.nih.gov/
FY12 appropriation: $338M (FY13: $319M) (20th/24, established 2000)
Mission: http://www.nibib.nih.gov/about-nibib
Funding decisions: http://www.nibib.nih.gov/funding/funding-policies

To address the potential interruption in funding for the first renewal of a new investigator's first R01 grant, the NIBIB has established a bridge funding policy for applications that are close to the funding payline. In addition, recognizing the concern that NIH peer review and funding practices often tend to favor more conservative research, the NIBIB sets as a goal to fund two or more RO1 applications that fit this scenario as select pay applications.

Funding Trends
- FY12 overall success rate (all mechanisms): 12.1%
- FY12 RPG success rate: 10.8% (new), 29.7% (renewal), 100% (supplement)
- FY12 RO1 success rate: 11.4% (new), 29.5% (renewal), 100% (supplement)

Additional Resources
- Resources for researchers: http://www.nibib.nih.gov/Research/Resources

Eunice Kennedy Shriver National Institute of Child Health and Human Development (NICHD)

Web site: http://www.nichd.nih.gov/
FY12 appropriation: $1.3B (FY13: $1.2B) (8th/24, established 1962)
Mission: http://www.nichd.nih.gov/about/overview/mission/Pages/index.aspx
Funding decisions: http://www.nichd.nih.gov/funding/strategies_concepts/index.cfm

In addition to standard funding policy for new and ESI applicants, RO1 and RO1-equivalent applications submitted by new investigators supported by NICHD Career Development (K) Awards are given special consideration.

Funding Trends
- FY12 overall success rate (all mechanisms): 12.5%
- FY12 RPG success rate: 11.1% (new), 32.9% (renewal), 12.5% (supplement)
- FY12 RO1 success rate: 11.3% (new), 31.0% (renewal), 20.0% (supplement)

Additional Resources
- Scientific resources: http://www.nichd.nih.gov/research/resources/Pages/index.aspx

National Institute of Deafness and Other Communication Disorders (NIDCD)

Web site: http://www.nidcd.nih.gov/

FY12 appropriation: $416M (FY13: $392M) (17th/24, established 1988)

Mission: http://www.nidcd.nih.gov/about/learn/pages/mission.aspx#1

Funding decisions: http://www.nidcd.nih.gov/funding/Pages/Default. aspx (see Funding Policy for current fiscal year)

The NIDCD allocates the majority of its RPG funds to applications in ranked (percentile or priority score) order. However, a portion of the funds is reserved for projects that may be outside this range but are of particular programmatic interest to the Institute.

Funding Trends

- Does not participate in the R03 parent announcement
- FY12 overall success rate (all mechanisms): 26.6%
- FY12 RPG success rate: 23.2% (new), 42.9% (renewal), 25.0% (supplement)
- FY12 R01 success rate: 22.8% (new), 43.6% (renewal), 25.0% (supplement)

Additional Resources

- Launching Your NIDCD Research Career: http://www.nidcd.nih.gov/ research/Pages/Launching-Your-NIDCD-Research-Career.aspx

National Institute of Dental and Craniofacial Research (NIDCR)

Web site: http://www.nidcr.nih.gov/

FY12 appropriation: $410M (FY13: $387M) (18th/24, established 1948)

Mission: http://www.nidcr.nih.gov/AboutUs/MissionandStrategicPlan/ MissionStatement/

Funding decisions: http://www.nidcr.nih.gov/grantsandfunding/ (scroll to NIDCR's Fiscal Plan for the current fiscal year)

The NIDCR provides individual consideration to all applications. As the fiscal year progresses, the Institute adjusts its plans to accommodate changes in the projected number of applications, the scientific merit of applications as reflected in the scores assigned during peer review, projected award costs, new scientific opportunities, and other relevant factors.

Funding Trends
- Does not participate in the R03 parent announcement
- FY12 overall success rate (all mechanisms): 21.2%
- FY12 RPG success rate: 20.7% (new), 37.8% (renewal), 100% (supplement)
- FY12 R01 success rate: 15.7% (new), 35.1% (renewal)

Additional Resources
- Clinical Research Toolkit: http://nidcr.nih.gov/research/toolkit

National Institute of Diabetes and Digestive and Kidney Disease (NIDDK)

Web site: http://www.niddk.nih.gov/
FY12 appropriation: $1.95B (FY13: $1.83B) (5th/24, established 1950)
Mission: http://www.nih.gov/about/almanac/organization/NIDDK.htm#mission
Funding decisions: http://www2.niddk.nih.gov/Funding/Grants/FundingPolicy.htm

Most R01 applications with a primary assignment to the NIDDK that request less than $500,000 direct costs per year and score at or better than the stated payline will receive an award (applications that have the NIDDK as a secondary assignment do not benefit from this payline). R01 applications requesting $500,000 or more in direct costs for any year will be held to a more stringent payline for both Type 1 and 2 applications. The NIDDK will exercise discretion and consider portfolio balance, programmatic importance, and other factors in determining which applications are awarded.

The NIDDK has a payline that is 2 percentile points more generous for new PIs and 5 percentile points more generous for ESI applicants. In addition, if a new investigator's R01 application is within 10 percentile points of the payline, it will receive enhanced second-level review for a reduced budget R01 or for an R56.

Similarly, if a competing renewal application falls near but beyond the nominal payline, the NIDDK will consider interim support on a case-by-case basis and provide limited support in selected cases. The goal is to preserve essential research resources pending the re-review of a revised application.

The NIDDK can choose to award a 1- or 2-year R56 grant to an R01 application scored outside the payline. These awards provide support for investigators to collect preliminary data and use these data to revise and improve their R01 applications.

Funding Trends
- Does not participate in the R03 or R21 parent announcements
- FY12 overall success rate (all mechanisms): 19.8%
- FY12 RPG success rate: 15.7% (new), 42.3% (renewal), 0.0% (supplement)
- FY12 R01 success rate: 15.1% (new), 35.6% (renewal), 0.0% (supplement)
- http://www2.niddk.nih.gov/Funding/Grants/FundingTrendsandValues.htm
- For R01 funding trend, see Figure 2.5.

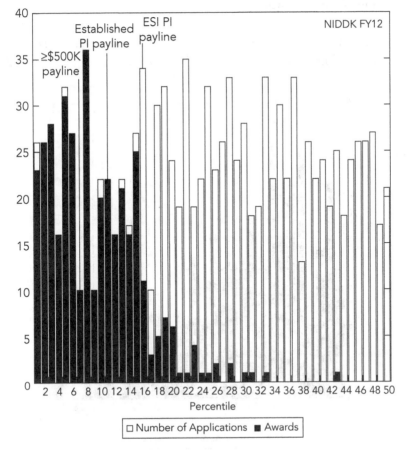

FIGURE 2.5 National Institute of Diabetes and Digestive and Kidney Disease: number of R01 applications versus awards, FY2012.

Additional Resources

- Resources for researchers: http://www2.niddk.nih.gov/Research/ Resources/
- Applicant guidelines (specific mechanisms): http://www2.niddk.nih. gov/Funding/Grants/ApplicantGuidelines/

National Institute on Drug Abuse (NIDA)

Web site: http://www.drugabuse.gov/
FY12 appropriation: $1.05B (FY13: $993M) (10th/24, established 1974)
Mission: http://www.drugabuse.gov/about-nida
Funding decisions:
http://www.drugabuse.gov/funding/funding-priorities/
    nida-funding-strategy

POs within a funding unit assess the slate of applications assigned to them in the context of the current grant portfolio and program priorities and provide

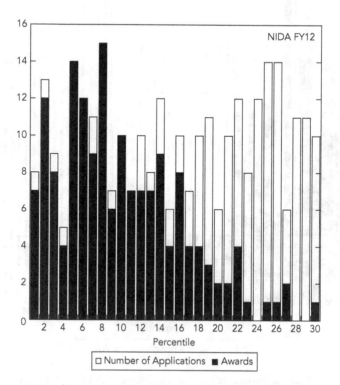

FIGURE 2.6 National Institute on Drug Abuse: number of R01 applications versus awards, FY2012.

recommendations to their Branch Chief, who in turn presents recommendations to the Division Director. These discussions occur on or about the time Council meets, and the comments and recommendations of Council members are also considered in the funding process. Senior staff in each unit participate in "shoplist" meetings attended by the Director and Deputy Director, Budget Office staff, and Grants Management staff at which they discuss each Division's prioritized list of applications as well as mitigating factors, such as whether an applicant is an ESI or new investigator; whether the application represents the only source of support available to the investigator; the scientific focus; whether the research is innovative or of high potential impact; and how much other research is already supported in the general area of the application. Based on these deliberations, a prioritized list of applications is determined.

Applications are paid in program priority order based on funds allocated for that Council funding cycle. Applications that are relatively high on the priority list but could not be funded are considered for possible funding later in the fiscal year, if more funds are made available in the final appropriation. (Chapter 5 discusses why the final appropriation is often not passed by Congress until after the first and sometimes second Council meetings.) While the Institute does not set a strict "payline," the scientific merit and potential impact, along with the application's priority (and percentile) score, weigh heavily in prioritizing applications and in making funding decisions.

Funding Trends

- FY12 overall success rate (all mechanisms): 21.2%
- FY12 RPG success rate: 20.3% (new), 30.4% (renewal), 20.0% (supplement)
- FY12 R01 success rate: 19.0% (new), 27.1% (renewal), 20.0% (supplement)
- For R01 funding trend, see Figure 2.6.

Additional Resources

- Research training and career development: http://www.drugabuse.gov/funding/research-training

National Institute of Environmental Health Sciences (NIEHS)

Web site: http://www.niehs.nih.gov
FY12 appropriation: $685M (FY13: $646M) (11th/24, established 1969)
Mission: http://www.niehs.nih.gov/about/index.cfm
Funding decisions: http://www.niehs.nih.gov/funding/grants/priorities/strategies/index.cfm

The NIEHS makes its funding decisions based on scientific merit, program balance, responsiveness to the Institute's priorities, and availability of funds. Although there are no formal procedures for new and ESI applicants, their applications are given priority when making funding decisions. Each year, following the appropriation of funds, an operating plan is developed that takes into account set-asides for specific initiatives and allocations for investigator-initiated applications. This plan applies primarily to RPGs (R01, R37, R15, R21, R55, R03, P01, U01), as other mechanisms (e.g., Centers) are considered on a program-by-program or case-by-case basis.

Funding Trends

- FY12 overall success rate (all mechanisms): 14.7%
- FY12 RPG success rate: 13.5% (new), 32.1% (renewal), 0% (supplement)
- FY12 R01 success rate: 11.2% (new), 32.9% (renewal), 0% (supplement)
- For R01 funding trend, see Figure 2.7.

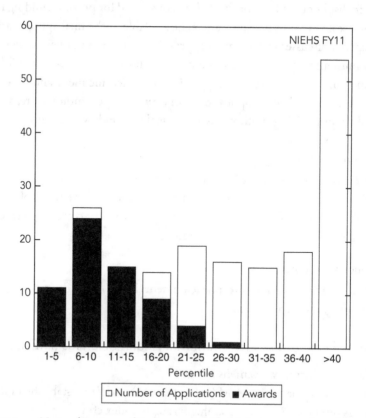

FIGURE 2.7 National Institute of Environmental Health Sciences: number of R01 applications versus awards, FY2011.

Additional Resources

- Resources for scientists: http://www.niehs.nih.gov/research/resources/index.cfm
- Funded research: http://tools.niehs.nih.gov/portfolio/

National Institute of General Medical Sciences Sciences (NIGMS)

Web site: http://www.nigms.nih.gov
FY12 appropriation: $2.4B (FY13: $2.3B) (4th/24, established 1962)
Funding decisions: http://www.nigms.nih.gov/Research/Policies.htm

Each National Advisory General Medical Sciences Council is assigned a set of applications from the most recent round of study sections (>1,000 total per Council meeting). Council members read the summary statements for these applications, providing a general check on the quality of the first level of peer review and advising program staff if they find cases where the comments and scores do not appear to be in good alignment. Most applications pass through this second level of review without specific comment, with Council concurring with the bulk of study section recommendations en bloc.

After a Council meeting, each NIGMS unit holds paylist meetings attended by POs at which applications are discussed and prioritized, beginning with the top-scoring applications. These applications (typically up to about half of the number that are expected to be funded) are given highest priority unless there are specific issues, such as those related to the NIGMS well-funded laboratory policy (http://www.nigms.nih.gov/Research/Application/NAGMSCouncilGuidelines.htm) or concerns raised at the Council meeting.

The discussion then turns to applications in the "gray area," typically extending to about 10 percentile points beyond what would be expected to be funded if all applications were awarded in straight percentile order. Each application is discussed, typically in percentile order, although sometimes applications from ESIs are discussed first. Consideration is given to whether the applicant is an ESI or new investigator, how much other support the applicant has (particularly if the application represents the only support available to the investigator), whether the Council has given specific advice on the application, whether the scientific area is perceived to be particularly exciting, and how much other research the NIGMS already supports in that general area. The other members of the unit listen to each PO's presentations, and the group then produces a prioritized list of applications.

Paylists are then developed using the prioritized lists, with budget adjustments for each application based on NIH- and NIGMS-wide policies as well as considerations specific to the application provided by the responsible program director. Applications are paid until the available funds are exhausted. Applications that are relatively high on the priority list but could not be funded with a given allocation are flagged for consideration later in the fiscal year, when more funds may become available.

Funding Trends

- Does not participate in the R03 or R21 parent announcements
- http://www.nigms.nih.gov/Research/trends.htm

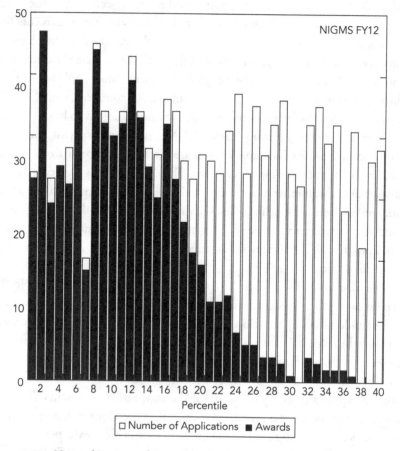

FIGURE 2.8 National Institute of General Medical Sciences: number of R01 applications versus awards, FY2012.

- FY12 overall success rate (all mechanisms): 24.4%
- FY12 RPG success rate: 17.9% (new), 42.6% (renewal), 33.3% (supplement)
- FY12 Ro1 success rate: 18.2% (new), 41.6% (renewal), 33.3% (supplement)
- http://www.nigms.nih.gov/Research/trends.htm
- For Ro1 funding trend, see Figure 2.8.

Additional Resources
- NIGMS feedback loop (blog): https://loop.nigms.nih.gov
- Research resources: http://www.nigms.nih.gov/Research/ResearchResources.htm

National Institute of Mental Health (NIMH)

Web site: http://www.nihm.nih.gov
FY12 appropriation: $1.5B (FY13: $1.4B) (7th/24, established 1949)
Mission: http://www.nimh.nih.gov/about/index.shtml
Funding decisions: http://www.nimh.nih.gov/funding/index.shtml
  (scroll down to Funding Strategy for Research Grants for current fiscal year)

While NIMH does not have a specific pay line, the Institute expects to support at least three-quarters of the applications with scores under the 20th percentile. NIMH will support sufficient applications from ESIs to ensure their success rate is equivalent to established investigators. Funding decisions are generally made in priority score or percentile order. Final funding decisions are based on alignment with the Strategic Plan, consideration of program relevance, commitment toward funding ESIs, availability of funds, and recommendations from the National Advisory Mental Health Council. Future year commitments for competing grant awards may be adjusted to reduce the number of out-year commitments.

Funding Trends
- http://www.nimh.nih.gov/research-funding/inside-nimh/2012-autumn-inside-nimh.shtml (check recent edition for latest FY trends)
- FY12 overall success rate (all mechanisms): 21.6%
- FY12 RPG success rate: 20.2% (new), 38.8% (renewal), 25.0% (supplement)
- FY12 Ro1 success rate: 20.8% (new), 37.6% (renewal), 27.3% (supplement)
- For Ro1 funding trend, see Figure 2.9.

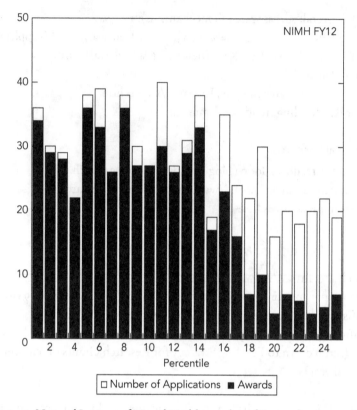

FIGURE 2.9 National Institute of Mental Health: number of R01 applications versus awards, FY2012.

Additional Resources

- Research resources: http://www.nimh.nih.gov/research-funding/grants/research-resources.shtml

National Institute of Minority Health and Health Disparities (NIMHD)

Web site: http://www.nimhd.nih.gov
FY12 appropriation: $276M (FY13: $260M) (21st/24, established in 1993 as NCMHD)
Mission: http://www.nimhd.nih.gov/about_ncmhd/mission.asp

Funding Trends

- Does not participate in the R01, R03, or R21 parent announcements
- FY12 overall success rate (all mechanisms): 9.9%

- FY12 RPG success rate: 9.9% (new)
- FY12 R01 success rate: 10.3% (new)

Additional Resources

- Programs: http://www.nimhd.nih.gov/our_programs/programs.asp

National Institute of Neurological Disorders and Stroke (NINDS)

Web site: http://www.ninds.nih.gov
FY12 appropriation: $1.6B (FY13: $1.5B) (6th/24, established 1950)
Mission: http://www.ninds.nih.gov/about_ninds/mission.htm
Funding decisions: http://www.ninds.nih.gov/funding/ninds_funding_
strategy.htm

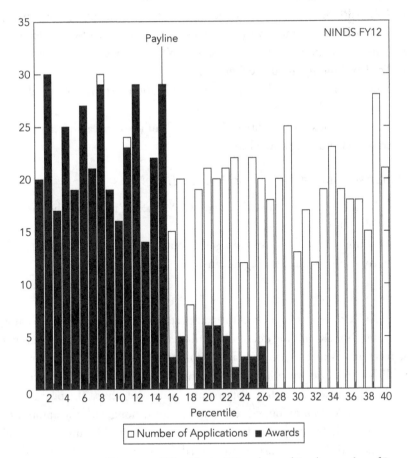

FIGURE 2.10 National Institute of Neurological Disorders and Stroke: number of R01 applications versus awards, FY2012.

A subset of applications that have percentiles within ten points of the current payline may be identified for high program priority consideration and funded on a case-by-case basis (all of these applications are considered by the NINDS Council). To maintain an average award length of 4 years, the NINDS will award 4 years of support for many applications that requested and were recommended for 5 years. A limited number of 5-year awards will be approved based on percentile rank of application, type of research (e.g. longitudinal studies and clinical trials may require 5 years to be completed), and new investigator status of applicant. The NINDS Advisory Council may recommend that a small subset of outstanding competing R01 applications be issued as Javits awards (http://www.ninds.nih.gov/research/epilepsyweb/javits.htm).

Funding Trends

- FY12 overall success rate (all mechanisms): 21.1%
- FY12 RPG success rate: 17.0% (new), 39.1% (renewal), 33.3% (supplement)
- FY12 R01 success rate: 17.1% (new), 38.2% (renewal), 50.0% (supplement)
- http://www.ninds.nih.gov/funding/2011-NINDS-Funding-Outcomes.htm
- For R01 funding trend, see Figure 2.10.
- How to write a research project grant application: http://www.ninds.nih.gov/funding/write_grant_doc.htm
- Resources for scientists: http://www.ninds.nih.gov/research/scientific_resources/index_research.htm

National Institute of Nursing Research (NINR)

FY12 appropriation: $145M (FY13: $136M) (22nd/24, established as NCNR in 1986)
Mission: https://www.ninr.nih.gov/aboutninr/ninr-mission-and-strategic-plan

Funding Decisions

The NINR does not publish a formal, predetermined payline for funding decisions. NINR funding decisions are driven by the science, by the number of meritorious investigator-initiated applications submitted in response to published strategic priorities, and through applications submitted in response to NINR-sponsored funding opportunity announcements. The peer review process and Advisory Council recommendations, along with the amount of funds available for new awards, determine the "payline" in any given fiscal year. The NINR does consider additional factors in making funding decisions, such as the science area, how innovative the research is, or whether the investigator is new or early stage.

Funding Trends

- Does not participate in the R03 parent announcement
- FY12 overall success rate (all mechanisms): 13.0%
- FY12 RPG success rate: 13.0% (new), 16.7% (renewal), 0% (supplement)
- FY12 R01 success rate: 14.5% (new), 16.7% (renewal), 0% (supplement)

Additional Resources

- Grantsmanship videos: http://www.ninr.nih.gov/Training/Grantsmanship.htm
- Grants development course: http://www.ninr.nih.gov/training/online-developing-nurse-scientists (must register first)
- Funded research: http://www.ninr.nih.gov/ResearchAndFunding/FundedNinrGrantsCollaborativeActivities/

National Library of Medicine (NLM)

Web site: http://www.nlm.nih.gov
FY12 appropriation: $346M (FY13: $318) (19th/24, established in 1956)
Mission: http://www.nlm.nih.gov/about/functstatement.html
Funding decisions: http://www.nlm.nih.gov/ep/Payplan.html

Funding decisions for RPG grants give weight to innovation in the informatics science, as well as significance and impact; the NLM expects the proposed work to have use case(s) in a biomedical domain and be generalizable beyond the use case. The NLM uses priority score and not percentile as one basis for pay decisions, coupled with mission relevance and innovation; the score range is published each year. Some projects that fall below the published payable range but are identified by staff or reviewers as "high-risk, high-reward" or highly innovative are taken to the Board of Regents Extramural Programs subcommittee for discussion and early concurrence voting. The NLM rarely selects an application with a secondary assignment for funding. Final award decisions reflect considerations of program relevance, portfolio balance, recommendations of the NLM Board of Regents, and availability of funds.

The NLM reviews about 80% of its own research project grants and all of its K awards; all grants are assigned to the Biomedical Library and Informatics Review Committee (BLIRC) or NLM Special Emphasis Panels (SEPs). The NLM has two unique activity codes (G grants), one used for nonrenewable support of information resource and one for scholarly book projects. The

NLM invests between 25% and 30% of its grant funds into pre- and postdoctoral training and career transition support for new researchers in biomedical informatics.

Funding Trends

- Does not participate in the R03 parent announcement
- FY12 overall success rate (all mechanisms): 16.1%
- FY12 RPG success rate: 12.8% (new), 12.5% (renewal)
- FY12 R01 success rate: 14.2% (new), 12.5% (renewal)

Additional Resources

- Programs: http://www.nlm.nih.gov/grants.html
- Funded research: http://www.nlm.nih.gov/ep/funded.html

John E. Fogarty International Center for the Advanced Study in the Health Sciences (FIC)

Web site: http://www.fic.nih.gov/
FY12 appropriation: $69.6M (FY13: $66.6M) (24th/24, established 1968)
Mission: http://www.fic.nih.gov/About/Pages/mission-vision.aspx
Funding decisions: http://www.fic.nih.gov/About/FundingStrategy/
    Pages/default.aspx

Funding decisions take into account program relevance and overall portfolio consideration, including responsiveness to the FIC Strategic Plan.

Funding Trends

- Does not participate in any parent announcement
- Funding opportunities: http://www.fic.nih.gov/Funding/Pages/
  Fogarty-Funding-Opps.aspx
- FY12 overall success rate (all mechanisms): 16.0%
- FY12 RPG success rate: 16.1% (new), 0% (renewal)
- FY12 R01 success rate: 10.7% (new), 0% (renewal)

Additional Resources

- FIC programs: http://www.fic.nih.gov/Programs/Pages/default.aspx
  (indicates which programs are closed and will not be re-competed for
  funding—very useful in avoiding developing a project in an area that
  FIC has indicated it will not support)

- Funded research portfolio: http://www.fic.nih.gov/Grants/Search/Pages/default.aspx
- Managing an FIC award: http://www.fic.nih.gov/Grants/Pages/Manage.aspx

National Center for Advancing Translational Sciences (NCATS)

Web site: http://www.ncats.nih.gov
FY12 appropriation: $575M (FY13: $542M) (13th/24, established 2011)
Mission: http://www.ncats.nih.gov/about/mission.html

Individual consideration is given to each grant application. Final award decisions are based on a variety of criteria, including but not limited to scientific merit, program relevance and balance, responsiveness to the Center's priorities, and availability of funds.

Funding Trends
- Does not participate in the R01, R03, or R21 parent announcements
- Did not receive funding authority until FY12

Additional Resources
- NCATS programs and initiatives: http://www.ncats.nih.gov/about/program-index/program-index.html
- Cures Acceleration Network (CAN) Review Board: http://www.csr.nih.gov/Roster_proto/members.asp?cid=104171&Title=Cures+Acceleration+Network+Review+Board&ABBR=CANRB

National Center for Complementary and Alternative Medicine (NCCAM)

Web site: http://nccam.nih.gov
FY12 appropriation: $128M (FY13: $121M) (23rd/24, established 1998)
Mission: http://www.nccam.nih.gov/about/ataglance
Funding decisions: http://nccam.nih.gov/grants/strategy/past

In general, grants are funded in priority score or percentile order. Additional considerations include program relevance and need, strategic priorities, duplication of ongoing research, availability of funds, whether the applicant is new or ESI, and recommendations by the Advisory Council.

Funding Trends

- Does not participate in the R03 parent announcement
- FY12 overall success rate (all mechanisms): 9.5%
- FY12 RPG success rate: 9.4% (new), 0% (renewal), 33.3% (supplement)
- FY12 R01 success rate: 10.0% (new), 0% (renewal), 33.3% (supplement)

Additional Resources

- Research blog: http://nccam.nih.gov/research/blog
- Clinical research toolbox: http://nccam.nih.gov/grants/toolbox
- Funded grant policies and resources: http://nccam.nih.gov/grants/policies
- Funded research portfolio: http://nccam.nih.gov/research/extramural/awards

3

Center for Scientific Review and the Peer Review Process

THE CENTER FOR SCIENTIFIC REVIEW (CSR) has served as the portal for all NIH grant applications since 1946. In addition to receipt and referral, CSR manages the scientific review groups (SRGs), generally referred to as study sections, which evaluate about 70% of the applications submitted to the NIH. As described in Chapter 1, public law mandates a two-stage review process designed to ensure fair, independent, scientifically rigorous funding decisions beyond the reach of special interests and earmarks. Although those of you with a pile of unfunded applications may have doubts, overall, the process works well.

CSR receives almost 90,000 applications a year and recruits more than 20,000 experts from academic and research institutions and industry as well as the intramural program at the NIH to review investigator-initiated grant applications for all award types except those reviewed within Institutes and Centers (ICs) (see Appendix for review contacts at each IC): program project/center (P), cooperative agreement (U), training (T), and career development (K) mechanisms as well as contracts (N) and applications submitted in response to Requests for Applications (RFAs) (funding opportunities are explained in Chapter 4; mechanisms in Chapter 7). Some ICs also review their own fellowship (F) applications. The locus of review is stated in the funding announcement.

Whether your application is referred to CSR or your IC, the NIH staff member in charge of your application at this point is the Scientific Review Officer (SRO). SROs usually have a doctorate in the field that is the scientific focus of the review group and are often former researchers themselves. The SRO identifies and recruits reviewers, enforces review policies throughout the review process, manages application lists (including ranking based on preliminary and final impact scores), and prepares summary statements. The SRO enters impact scores electronically, after which percentiles are generated for each application appropriate for percentiling. You would interact with the SRO prior to the review, both to request appropriate reviewers (more on this later in the chapter and in Chapter 8) and to submit postsubmission application materials about 6 weeks prior to the study section meeting; NIH policy (currently, http://grants.nih.gov/grants/guide/notice-files/NOT-OD-13-030.html) and the SRO determine what can be submitted, how long and in what format supplemental materials should be (including videos, http://grants1.nih.gov/grants/guide/notice-files/NOT-OD-12-141.html), and when it must be received to be considered by reviewers.

The initial receipt and referral process is generally straightforward, but your application can be administratively returned for a variety of reasons, even if it made it through grants.gov, such as if your application lacks the required cover letter granting approval from your primary IC agreeing to accept the submission with a budget exceeding $500,000 (direct costs in any 1 year). Noncompliance with formatting restrictions, budget type (modular rather than detailed or vice versa, depending on where your application falls in relation to the $250,000 threshold), and requirements specific to the application will also result in your application being returned.

Another possible reason for return is the submission of a new application that is not substantially changed from a previously revised application that was not funded. Starting in 2009, to manage reviewer burden and increase the number of applications funded their first time in, the NIH limited applicants to two submissions (http://grants.nih.gov/grants/guide/notice-files/NOT-OD-09-003.html): a new application (A0) and one amendment (A1). The NIH checks for surreptitious "A2" applications (i.e., the revision of an unfunded A1) using software and manpower, and the ruling that an application is ineligible can be made at any stage of the review process.

As suggested by the NIH policy guidelines (http://grants.nih.gov/grants/policy/amendedapps.htm), you should discuss your new A0 aims with your Program Officer (PO) if you are not sure whether they have too much overlap with your unfunded A1; two-thirds of the aims must be new, and the research plan must be substantively changed. Alternatively, you can submit your project under a new mechanism (e.g., R21) or in response to an RFA (in the happy circumstance that one is issued that matches your science). However, you cannot simply move your R01 from one program announcement (PA) to another and have it considered "new" (A0), at least not without altering the aims and approach as just noted (more on this in Chapter 13).

The NIH has communicated their intention to maintain the policy change that eliminates A2 applications (http://nexus.od.nih.gov/all/2012/11/28/the-a2-resubmission-policy-continues-a-closer-look-at-recent-data/), despite concerns raised by investigators in the extramural research community, so you will want to factor this submission limitation into your long-term grant application strategy.

Getting back to CSR, the "referral" involves the assignment of your application to a primary IC, sometimes to a secondary IC, and to an SRG, all of which are in your control, to a certain extent. You can and should include a cover letter (an optional upload in the electronic SF424 package) with your application. You can request the IC(s) and study section to which you want the application assigned as well as those SRGs you do not want to review your proposal. You can also use the cover letter to list, by name, any individuals who should *not* serve as reviewers due to conflict of interest or competition as well as describe the type of expertise reviewers who are assigned to your application should have (in this case, no names, just the key disciplines/expertise). These requests are presented in bullet format, with a separate paragraph explaining the rationale for each (see also Chapter 8).

About 7 to 10 days after submission, your eRA Commons account will list in the Status section (List of Applications/Grants) your application identification number (http://www.niaid.nih.gov/researchfunding/glossary/pages/a.aspx#appno), which you should now use when communicating with anyone at the NIH about your proposal. The identification number indicates the type of application (new, renewal, supplement), the funding mechanism (e.g., R01, K08, T32), the primary IC, the unique project serial number, the funding year, and whether the application is amended or supplemental. For example:

1R01 CA1234567-01 A1

indicates that this is a new (Type 1) amended (A1) R01 application for project 1234567 at the National Cancer Institute (CA). Type 2 projects are competing renewals, while Type 3 projects are competitive supplements (Type 5 are non-competing renewals). When the NIH stopped permitting a second amended application, the "A2" suffix dropped from use.

Consider the import of this grant application number:

5R01 GM000091-62

which signifies 62 years of funding for the "Structure and Function of Enzymes—Role of Metals." Up to 46 of these years were funded by the National Institute of General Medical Sciences (NIGMS; established in 1962), whereas the award, which ended in 2008 (plus a no-cost extension into 2009), would have started in 1946—the year the Research Grants Office was created at the NIH. Remarkably, there was only one change of PI along the way.

You should not have any surprises with regard to the IC assignment. Your PO will not refuse to accept assignment of an application you have discussed in advance with him or her (Chapters 2 and 10), but if you did not request a specific IC, and the primary assignment was not obvious based on your abstract and specific aims (e.g., if the application might be of interest to multiple ICs), you might find yourself at a different IC than you expected. If you have any questions about the IC to which your application has been assigned (including dual assignment), you should communicate with the assigned PO.

When you click on the Application ID link in your eRA Commons account, you will first see the IRG to which your application was referred and shortly thereafter the specific SRG (usually within 2 weeks of submission).

If you have any concerns about the SRG assignment, you should contact the SRO of the study section to which your application was assigned to inquire why your request was not honored and whether the application can be moved to your preferred group. The SROs of your assigned and your requested study sections likely discussed the matter during the referral of your application, and often their insight (not something you can discern by reading SRG descriptions and rosters) will result in your receiving a better review than if you had insisted on going to your requested study section. If you are still concerned about the roster, you can inquire if the SRO could add ad hoc members appropriate for your science. You could also contact the chief of the IRG for advice, though you should be able to work things out with the SROs. No matter whom you contact, you will need an objective rationale for moving your application based on the science rather than your preference for a "friendly" panel.

You may discover that your application was assigned to a Special Emphasis Panel (SEP), either due to the nature of the funding opportunity or to a member conflict with your application. In the past, some applicants would try to game the system to get assigned to a SEP, which traditionally was smaller and might be tailored to just one or two applications. Due to budget constraints, however, CSR is empaneling fewer and broader SEPs covering more diverse topics and expertise, so this assignment no longer necessarily provides a strategic, friendly edge.

You will have known from the outset, based on the funding mechanism or opportunity, whether your application would be going to an IC-specific SRG or SEP. If you unexpectedly find yourself at a study section managed by the IC rather than CSR (or vice versa), you can again contact the SRO or, in this case, your PO (since it is within the same IC), for advice (or reassurance).

Picking the Right Reviewers

Although public law dictates the basic peer review framework (http://www.gpo.gov/fdsys/search/pagedetails.action?browsePath=Title+42%2FChapter+I%2FSubchapter+D%2FPart+52h&granuleId=CFR-2007-title42-vol1-part52h&packageId=CFR-2007-title42-vol1&collapse=true&fromBrowse=true), CSR continually monitors how the review process is implemented and works to "enhance" peer review efficiency and efficacy. The Center adjusts study section alignment as needed to keep up with evolving scientific disciplines and technologies and has restructured the application and review process to minimize burden and the time between application and award.

In fact, CSR systematically evaluates IRGs, the umbrella organizations under which study sections in the same scientific field are clustered, on a biannual basis. Recommendations from advisory groups may result in the creation, modification, or elimination of study sections (http://public.csr.nih.gov/aboutcsr/CSROrganization/Pages/NewReorganization.aspx). Overlap exists both among study sections in the same IRG and with those from different IRGs, so you should keep monitoring fluctuations in SRG descriptions and member rosters (http://public.csr.nih.gov/StudySections/Pages/default.aspx) to be sure the right people are reading your science. For example, you can check out the Tumor Microenvironment SRG (regular membership roster as well as rosters for each of the last three meetings) at the CSR Web site (see Fig. 3.1). You will also read (not shown in Figure 3.1) bullet points of topics covered and a list of closely related SRGs you might also want to consider.

You can also query RePORTER (http://projectreporter.nih.gov) to see what applications reviewed by standing CSR study sections receive funding. While study sections do not "fund" applications, any application receiving an award must have been scored well to receive consideration, and seeing what

Tumor Microenvironment Study Section [TME]

The Tumor Microenvironment [TME] Study Section reviews grant applications that deal with basic mechanisms of interactions between tumor and host system including stromal cells, extracellular matrix (ECM) and extracellular molecules. Emphasis is on evaluation of the tumor as an organ-like structure with complex, dynamic cross-talk. Studies of tumor-stroma interactions including cell-cell interaction, tumor induced alterations of ECM, tumor angiogenesis and lymphangiogenesis, and organ specific metastasis are assigned to this study section, with studies in animal models and more translational work in human cells.

Rosters

TME Membership Roster   TME Meeting Rosters

FIGURE 3.1   CSR Web site overview of the Tumor Microenvironment SRG (http://public.csr.nih.gov/StudySections/IntegratedReviewGroups/OBTIRG/TME/Pages/default.aspx). Not shown is a list of topics covered and related study sections.

research has secured funding gives you an idea of what is of most interest to a particular panel. Members of the SRG often go back themselves to search RePORTER to see whether "their applications"—the ones they were most enthusiastic about being funded—did in fact receive awards.

For example, see the search results for currently funded Type 1 (new) and Type 2 (competing renewal) applications reviewed by the Tumor Microenvironment SRG in Figure 3.2.

Project Search Results

Back to Query Form   Save Query   Share Query

Export All Projects

T Act	Project	Year	Sub #	Project Title	Contact PI / Project Leader	Organization	FY	Admin IC	Funding IC	FY Total Cost by IC	Similar Projects
2 R01	CA113451	06A1		3D-ADHESION STROMAGENESIS IN CANCER PERMISSIVENESS	CUKIERMAN, EDNA	INSTITUTE FOR CANCER RESEARCH	2012	NCI	NCI	$245,775	
1 R01	CA166473	01		A NOVEL PLASMINOGEN RECEPTOR IN BREAST CANCER	MUELLER, BARBARA MARIA et al.	TORREY PINES INST FOR MOLECULAR STUDIES	2012	NCI	NCI	$464,971	
1 R21	CA164322	01		A TRANSLATIONAL MODEL OF EVOLUTION OF MYELOMA ADHESION-MEDIATED DRUG RESISTANCE	SILVA, ARIOSTO S	H. LEE MOFFITT CANCER CTR & RES INST	2012	NCI	NCI	$235,401	
1 R01	CA160890	01A1		ADRENERGIC REGULATION OF TUMOR INFLAMMATION AND METASTATIC DISSEMINATION	SLOAN, ERICA KATE	UNIVERSITY OF CALIFORNIA LOS ANGELES	2012	NCI	NCI	$319,560	
1 R01	CA164122	01A1		B7-H1 SIGNALING IN OVARIAN CANCER	CURIEL, TYLER J.	UNIV OF TX HSC, SA	2012	NCI	NCI	$310,040	
1 R01	CA193562	01A1		BONE MARROW MSCS/PERICYTES: GATEKEEPERS CONTROLLING SKELETAL METASTASIS	CAPLAN, ARNOLD I.	CASE WESTERN RESERVE UNIVERSITY	2012	NCI	NCI	$315,367	
1 R21	CA164232	01		CD147 BIOLOGICAL FUNCTION AND ROLE AS A BIOMARKER OF MGUS TO MYELOMA PROGRESSION	JELINEK, DIANE F	MAYO CLINIC	2012	NCI	NCI	$171,499	
1 R01	CA154728	01A1		CELL-SPECIFIC TRANSCRIPTION IN CANCER MICROENVIRONMENT IN VITRO AND IN VIVO	STEINMAN, RICHARD A	UNIVERSITY OF PITTSBURGH AT PITTSBURGH	2012	NCI	NCI	$323,753	

FIGURE 3.2   RePORTER (http://projectreporter.nih.gov/reporter.cfm) allows you to search funded awards by study section to review the types of projects receiving competitive scores by the SRG you are targeting.

You will need to identify your study sections through the CSR Web site before turning to RePORTER, since some panels have different composition and foci but essentially the same or similar sounding names (see Figure 3.3).

You should also poll your mentors and colleagues regarding their experiences with specific study sections. While your application may not be appropriate for their "favorite" panels, you may get insight into which groups to consider or avoid. Similarly, your PO likely attends various study section meetings in your field and can give advice as to how your application might fare in the hands of one group versus another. You can likewise ask the SROs of study sections you are considering whether they feel your science is appropriate for their reviewers.

Once you have the application in what you hope are the right hands, there is not much more you can do. In the past, applicants could submit new data just prior to the review, but now the postsubmission materials are quite limited (at the time of this writing, http://grants.nih.gov/grants/policy/nihgps_2012/nihgps_ch2.htm#post_submission_materials), though potentially useful, if you do not want to wait a cycle until a manuscript under review has been published. You can send allowable postsubmission information, including news of

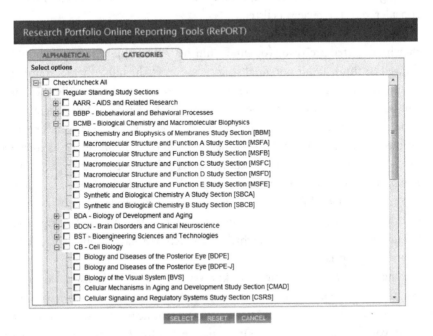

FIGURE 3.3 RePORTER only lists SRG names and abbreviations, so be sure to do your research at the CSR Web site (http://public.csr.nih.gov/StudySections/Pages/default.aspx) first to distinguish between similarly named study sections.

a manuscript accepted for publication (but not the manuscript itself), to the SRO at least 30 days prior to the SRG meeting date. The SRO will often contact applicants about 2 months prior to when the study section meets and indicate what is and is not allowable (some FOAs allow specific additional materials) and the format and timing for submission. Any postsubmission material must be sent with the concurrence (not just a "cc" on your e-mail message) of your Authorized Organizational Representative (or Signing Official), generally the director of your sponsored programs office or someone in the office of research—the person who signed off on the submission of the application itself.

It is not until a month or so before the SRG meets (often only a couple of weeks in advance of a SEP meeting) that you will be able to see the final roster. If you see a competitor or someone else with a conflict of interest whom you did not anticipate and whom you do not believe can be impartial, or you do not see anyone with the appropriate expertise to appreciate your science listed for that meeting, you can contact the SRO with your concerns. However, the rationale must be objective and compelling—more than the reviewer being unkind at a poster session or based on an assumption that the reviewer rejected a manuscript. In addition, doing so at this point may mean waiting a cycle to be reviewed, if you did not want your application to be considered by the reviewers listed.

Although most investigators think about their SRG assignment only after they have started preparing (or almost finished) their application, you would do well to think about potential study sections at the outset, when framing your aims and approach, and tailor your proposal accordingly, while you can still be flexible in doing so. Look at the research of regular SRG members and talk with colleagues to get an idea of how to meet these reviewers' expectations and take into account their perspectives of and contributions to the field. Writing to a very specific audience may allow you to save space otherwise needed to convince them of the significance of your work and allow you to reprioritize this space to convincing them you have the best research team to achieve compelling scientific aims of mutual interest. You can also be sure to address concepts on which SRG members have published and cite them as appropriate.

One thing *not* to do once you know where your application has been assigned is to discuss (or even mention) your application to any reviewers on the study section, even in social settings or at scientific meetings. On the other hand, you do want to be sure your science gets in front of these reviewers, so be sure to present (posters if not invited for an oral presentation) at meetings they attend, particularly if your work crosses various fields. This could be you or your postdoc or graduate student, though be sure they know not to talk with anyone specifically about a pending application. When selecting outside speakers for your department or center seminar series, consider inviting those who are shaping funding decisions to get their take on what is important in the field, now and in the future. Again, do not bring up any specific proposals you are planning or have already submitted for review.

How Your Application Is Reviewed

Although what goes on in the minds of your assigned reviewers is not transparent, the review process to which they must adhere is. CSR has created excellent videos to help applicants prepare competitive applications, understand the review process, and observe a study section meeting (http:// public.csr.nih.gov/ApplicantResources/Pages/default.aspx). You can look at the review criteria for components common to all applications (http://public. csr.nih.gov/ReviewerResources/GeneralReviewGuidelines/Pages/default. aspx) and specific to each type of application reviewed (http://public.csr.nih. gov/ReviewerResources/SpecificReviewGuidelines/Pages/default.aspx).

You can also read the instructions and advice given to new study section members and new study section chairs, which might round out your overall feel for how these meetings unfold. One thing to remember is that the NIH takes confidentiality and conflict of interest very seriously (http://grants.nih. gov/grants/peer/COI_Information.pdf); you should not dwell on a concern that reviewers might steal your science or alert your competitors. You should also be aware that your friends on the study section may need to declare a conflict of interest if they have mentored or collaborated with you in the past 5 years. Another point to keep in mind is that only reviewers who attend the full meeting (not necessarily everyone listed on the roster) contribute to the final impact scores. Of course, you must not assume that all the reviewers who attend the full meeting will have read your application—this is not a prerequisite for assigning an impact score.

Briefly, your primary and secondary reviewers plus at least one additional reader will be selected by the SRO based on their having expertise relevant to your proposed work. You should not assume the other members of the study section will be familiar with your science. Your assigned reviewers read your application thoroughly, write a critique before the meeting, and assign preliminary scores for each review criterion as well as an initial overall impact score.

The initial impact scores determine which applications will be discussed at the meeting and the order in which they will be reviewed (best, and therefore lowest, scores first). In addition, applications from new and early stage investigator applicants are discussed as a group first (in ascending order of preliminary score), then applications from established investigators. The preliminary scores and comments for each application are available to all study section members less than a week before the meeting; reviewers are encouraged to read the comments of their peers in advance of the meeting, and most do. The proposed order of review is sent out a few days in advance, and exceptions to the proposed list of applications for discussion are decided at the beginning of the meeting. Generally, the bottom half of submissions are triaged (also called streamlined) and not discussed unless a reviewer on the committee specifically requests that an otherwise triaged application be discussed.

If your application is discussed:

- First, any reviewers in conflict are asked to leave the room.
- Next, the Chair asks the primary reviewer, the secondary reviewer, and the reader to give their preliminary impact scores, which sets the tone for the discussion, particularly if the reviewers have widely divergent scores.
- Your primary reviewer presents your application and summarizes its strengths and weaknesses; the other assigned reviewers then add their comments (mainly those in disagreement, as they are asked not to repeat points with which they agree).
- At this point, your application is open for group discussion.
- When the discussion is drawn to a close, your assigned reviewers give their final impact scores, which set the "scoring range" for other eligible SRG members, who must indicate if they are giving a score outside this range. For example, if your assigned reviewers gave scores of 2 and 3, anyone else on the study section who wanted to assign a score of 1 or 4 (or higher) would need to explain why.

Alternatively, your application may undergo review via an Internet-Assisted Meeting (IAM) (formerly known as Asynchronous Electronic Discussion) (http://public.csr.nih.gov/ReviewerResources/ToolsAndTechnology/Pages/Internet-Assisted-Meeting-(IAM)-Overview.aspx), in which case there is no meeting—and no body language or live discussion. Instead, preliminary scores are made available to all reviewers via the Internet

Assisted Review section of each reviewer's eRA Commons account, and the "discussion" then occurs via threaded messages at a separate IAM Web site. This is where assigned reviewers provide introductory comments about the application (the primary reviewer summarizes the approach in two to three sentences). Study section members can post questions and comments about each application as well as "discussion scores," which indicate the changing level of enthusiasm for an application. The discussion scores of assigned reviewers are used to establish the scoring range for an application. The study section Chair ensures that the discussion of each application is summarized appropriately prior to final scoring, and each study section member can provide a final score for all discussed applications for which they have no conflict.

While convenient in terms of reducing travel time and expense and accommodating reviewers across multiple time zones, these Internet reviews require study section members to log on several times a day over the course of a week, and critical communication via body language and live exchanges is lost (and cannot be observed by POs). However, you have no say in whether your application is reviewed at an in-person meeting or on the Internet, so do not include a request for a particular type of review in your cover letter (discussed earlier and in Chapter 8).

The key take-home message for you as a PI in considering the review process is how little time is devoted to each application discussed. You will spend hundreds of hours on your research and preparing the application, the primary reviewer will invest several hours evaluating the package, the secondary reviewer and reader will likely be less thorough, and the unassigned panel members will (hopefully) read your abstract and specific aims but not much else. The discussion—if your application makes it to that point—will last no more than 10–15 minutes.

Therefore, you should view your application as an elevator speech rather than a detailed protocol or a review article. You do not want to submit a solid block of full-justified text with minimal white space. You want to be kind to your reviewers, who are engaged in community service. Envision them trying to read your application at 2 a.m., between their own overdue manuscript reviews and a graduate student thesis, with a sick child wailing in the background. You do not want to make this task more difficult than necessary.

Your application should be visibly inviting to read and it should flow well (see Chapter 9), not forcing reviewers to back up to reread dense sentences full of abbreviations, acronyms, jargon, and shorthand references that might not be part of his or her lexicon. You want them to get excited about your application, which then becomes one of "their" applications, such that they want to see it discussed and funded.

You want to clearly make the point why the work is important to do and why you are the person or team to do it—that the research will do best "in your hands." This is what reviewers will want to know in assessing the overall impact—the "likelihood for [your] project to exert a sustained, powerful influence on the research field(s) involved."

To convince the entire study section, this means crafting the best possible specific aims page—the only page that might be read by everyone on the panel—so it very clearly makes your case and generates enthusiasm (see Chapter 8).

Keep in mind that your reviewer is essentially reading about the future. Make it exciting, a future he or she will want to see come to pass, results that he or she will want to read in a journal. As we noted earlier, reviewers often check RePORTER to see whether "their" applications received funding, and you want to inspire them to think of *your* application as one of "their" applications. You get there by selling them on yourself as an applicant and your science as solid (even if high-risk), compelling research.

You also get there by making the primary reviewer's job easy: organize the application to match the review criteria under consideration and provide talking points to help your primary reviewer convince the rest of the study section to make your application one they want to see funded. You must motivate your primary reviewer to advocate for your application, particularly if dissenting opinions are raised by the other reviewers or panel members.

One often-overlooked strategy for convincing the reviewer to become your advocate is to write in the first person (e.g., "We will…" or "Our aims are…" rather than "The goals are to…" or "The proposal aims to…"). You want the reviewer to begin to develop a relationship with you personally, rather than leave him or her with a generic-sounding, impersonal protocol. Writing in the first person shows confidence and sincerity rather than pomposity—so long as your claims are within reason.

Remember, too, that you are writing for the reviewer, not for you. Write what is important for the reviewer to know, not every tangential line of thought you find interesting, not in an attempt to impress the reviewer with your depth of knowledge (beyond what is needed to establish the significance of the work). Having colleagues not involved with your research read and critique your application should help you uncover what is missing or unclear. Listen to them and revise accordingly (more on this in Chapter 10).

What the Score (or Lack Thereof) Means

All reviewed applications receive a summary statement. All discussed applications receive an impact/priority score. You will find your impact/priority score in the Application Information column (middle of the third box down, farthest left column) on the Status Information page for your application in eRA Commons; the summary statement will be listed up in the upper right box under Other Relevant Documents. The layout of the screen is shown in Figure 3.4. Please note too that this screen shot illustrates that your eRA Commons status may lag behind reality, in that the status still indicates that the SRG review is pending, whereas a summary statement is available.

We will cover in Chapters 11 and 13 what to do if your application is not discussed or does not receive a fundable score, but here we will briefly review the criterion and overall impact scoring. As noted earlier, you will only receive an impact score if your application is discussed, but all applications receive the five criterion scores—Significance, Investigator(s), Innovation, Approach, and Environment—plus critiques by the assigned reviewers in the form of bulleted strengths and weaknesses.

Reviewers can also make additional comments to the applicant, including encouragement to resubmit or a recommendation to redirect his or her energies. CSR provides critique templates and examples for a variety of funding mechanisms, and you can view a sample R01 and R21 summary statement through NIAID (http://www.niaid.nih.gov/researchfunding/grant/Pages/appsamples.aspx).

With regard to the scores themselves, the NIH uses a 9-point scale in which lower is better and 5 is considered to be a "good medium-impact application" (see Figure 3.5).

Reviewers are encouraged to go back and revise their critiques following the discussion, but not all do, which is why some summary statements can be a bit puzzling. You must remember that the overall impact/priority score is not calculated from the individual criterion scores—again, there can often be an apparent disconnect between one reviewer's criterion scores and the final overall impact score assigned. This is where your PO, assuming he or she heard the discussion, can help clarify the key take-home points.

The SRO enters the reviewer's final impact scores, which the computer uses to generate the final overall impact/priority score for each discussed application by calculating the mean score from the impact scores assigned by all eligible study section members (those not in conflict who attended the entire meeting) and multiplying this by 10. The final overall impact score

General Grant Information

		Other Relevant Documents
Status:	Scientific Review Group review completed; Council review pending. Refer any questions to Program Official.	e-Application
Institution Name:	UNIVERSITY OF PITTSBURGH AT PITTSBURGH	Summary Statement
School Name:	SCHOOL OF MEDICINE	Additions for Review (0 documents)
School Category:	SCHOOLS OF MEDICINE	
Division Name:	NONE	
Department Name:	MEDICINE	Correspondence
PI Name:	WHITCOMB, DAVID Clement	Referral
Application ID:	2T32DK063922-11	Date Description Action
Proposal Title:	Digestive Diseases Training Program	
Last Status Update Date:	10/30/2012	
Proposal Receipt Date:	05/24/2012	
Current Award Notice Date:		
Application Source:	Grants.gov	
Project Period Begin Date:	07/01/2003	
Project Period End Date:	06/30/2018	
eApplication Status:	Submission Complete	
FOA:	[PA11-184] – RUTH L. KIRSCHSTEIN NATIONAL RESEARCH SERVICE AWARD (NRSA) INSTITUTIONAL RESEARCH TRAINING GRANTS (PARENT T32)	
NIH Appl. ID:	8474331	

Status History

Effective Date	Status Message
05/30/2012	Scientific Review Group review pending. Refer any questions to the Scientific Review Administrator.
05/24/2012	Application entered into system

Institute or Center Assignment

Institute or Center	Assignment Date
NATIONAL INSTITUTE OF DIABETES AND DIGESTIVE AND KIDNEY DISEASES (Primary)	05/24/2012
NATIONAL INSTITUTE OF DIABETES AND DIGESTIVE AND KIDNEY DISEASES (Primary)	05/30/2012

Application Information

		Study Section		Advisory Council(AC) Information	
Award Document Number:	TDK063922C	Scientific Review Group:	DDK-C	Meeting Date:	02/13/2013
FSR Accepted Code:	N	Council Meeting Date(YYYY/MM):	2013/01	Meeting Time:	08:30
Snap Indicator Code:		Meeting Date:	10/24/2012		
Impact/Priority Score:	20	Meeting Time:	06:00		
Percentile:		Study Roster:	View Meeting Roster		
Early Stage Investigator Eligible:					
New Investigator Eligible:					

FIGURE 3.4 When your application is reviewed, the eRA Commons application status page will list the impact/priority score and percentile (if applicable) under Application Information (bottom-most section) and a link to the summary statement under Other Relevant Documents (upper right section).

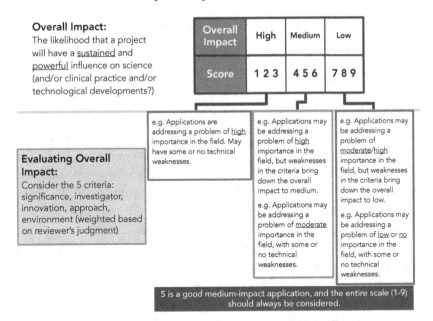

FIGURE 3.5 All review groups use the same 9-point scoring scale to assign individual criterion and overall impact scores.

ranges from 10 (high impact) through 90 (low impact) and is reported on the summary statement. Applications that are not discussed have ++ instead of a numerical score next to "SRG Action" on the face page of the summary statement.

An application may be designated as Not Recommended for Further Consideration (NRFC) if it lacks significant and substantial merit or presents serious ethical problems. These are identified at the outset of the study section meeting, and some may be rescued from this classification. If not, an NRFC application does not proceed further through the second level of review.

Percentiles versus Paylines versus Success Rate

Of these three concepts (percentile, payline, success rate), CSR is only responsible for calculating percentiles, which indicate the relative rank of your overall impact score among all the scores assigned by your SRG at its last three meetings. The SRO compares your overall impact score with a table of relative rankings of scores of applications reviewed during the past three study section meetings, which is used in the following formula:

$$(100 \div \text{no. of applications}) \times (\text{relative rank} - 0.5) = \text{percentile}$$

So, if your application was one of 119 applications submitted, and its overall impact score resulted in a relative rank of 38, the percentile would be:

$$(100 \div 119) \times (38 - 0.5) = 31.51 = 32\text{nd percentile}$$

The final value is rounded up to the next whole number and will fall in a range from 1 to 99, with lower numbers representing better scores. Percentiles are calculated for unsolicited R01 applications (those not submitted to an RFA) and other mechanisms for which that particular SRG reviews sufficient numbers of applications each cycle to support percentiling (e.g., F mechanisms, R21). In eRA Commons, posting of the percentile may lag behind the impact score.

You need to remember that percentiles are tied to your study section, not to your IC, and they change from cycle to cycle, so it is hard for you to even compare notes with peers whose applications were reviewed by the same group at a prior or later meeting. In addition, CSR periodically recalibrates the scoring and percentiling of applications to enforce "spreading" of scores to use the full range (versus clustering the majority of scores in the 10–30 range, because reviewers would like to see all these applications considered for funding).

Data shown in Chapter 2 allow you to compare the number of R01 applications considered for funding at each percentile compared with the number of awards made by many ICs at each percentile (and you will see the range of percentiles at which applications receive funding varies by IC). This represents the "pay range," the score or percentile range considered when creating "paylists" or setting a payline. Paylines, which are determined individually by each IC, are not always calculated formulaically, are not always publically available, and are not always numeric (i.e., not all ICs use a "hard" payline as a threshold for funding decisions). The payline at one IC should not be used to gauge the likelihood of funding for an application of the same mechanism at another IC.

Success rate is calculated based on the number of awards made in a specific fiscal year divided by the number of applications for a given activity code. Note that, due to a variety of factors, paylines and success rates are not directly comparable. The Office of Extramural Research presents these data cut in several ways in the NIH Research Portfolio Online Reporting Tools (RePORT) (http://report.nih.gov). You can find success rate broken down by IC, fiscal year, activity code, application type (new, renewal), amendment status, PI status (established, new/early stage investigator), and so on. RePORT includes a wealth of other data that could be useful in helping you plan your NIH application strategy (discussed in Chapter 6).

Getting back to percentiles, the intent of this calculation is to counter "score creep," in which reviewers assign lower and lower scores (i.e., better scores) to applications they merit as scientifically worthy when they observe IC paylines drop. Even if many applications receive a low score, the percentile indicates their relative rank over time. However, the data can still become skewed, as illustrated by the National Institute of Allergy and Infectious Diseases (http://www.niaid.nih.gov/researchfunding/grant/strategy/Pages/7payline.aspx#c). This is why many ICs, such as the NIGMS, do not set "hard" paylines but instead discuss applications within a competitive percentile range to create paylists. This is also why CSR recalibrates scores and percentiles periodically (http://public.csr.nih.gov/PolicyChanges/Pages/Notice-on-the-Recalibration-of-Percentiles.aspx).

The outcomes of the various approaches to funding decisions result in remarkably similar funding curves for different ICs as shown throughout Chapter 2 and in Chapter 12 (Figure 12.1).

Becoming a Reviewer

Reviewing grant applications is a community service, but one with major impact on the future of science in the United States. Reviewers shape the direction of biomedical research through their perspective on what constitutes the best science. The time commitment is significant, particularly since they should be working on their own grant applications at about the same time their reviews are due, and those who do a good job are often called upon by SROs to pitch in on other study sections.

The Center for Scientific Review is always looking for qualified reviewers. SROs find reviewers through the literature, scientific meetings, professional societies, current or past SRG members, recently funded PIs, POs, and Council members. You can also nominate yourself for consideration (http://public.csr.nih.gov/ReviewerResources/BecomeAReviewer/Pages/How-Scientists-Are-Selected.aspx#Process), either to be a regular member or part of the Early Career Reviewer Program (http://public.csr.nih.gov/ReviewerResources/BecomeAReviewer/Pages/Overview-of-ECR-program.aspx). While the major benefit is having a front-row seat to see how the review process works and which science is judged sufficiently meritorious for funding, you may also benefit from late and/or continuous submission of grant applications (http://public.csr. nih.gov/ReviewerResources/BecomeAReviewer/Pages/Benefits-of-Being-a-Reviewer.aspx).

Peer Review Resources

- CSR Peer Review Resources: http://public.csr.nih.gov/Pages/default.aspx
- OER Peer Review Policies: http://grants.nih.gov/grants/peer/peer.htm
- Search study sections by keyword: http://public.csr.nih.gov/ StudySections/Pages/default.aspx
- Rocket Boys: http://public.csr.nih.gov/aboutcsr/NewsAndPublications/ Outreach/Pages/default.aspx

4

Office of Extramural Research

ALTHOUGH EACH INSTITUTE AND CENTER (IC) has its own way of managing its funding and fiscal policy (Chapter 2), most aspects of the grant application and award process are common across the NIH, and these policies are administered by the Office of Extramural Research (OER), which is in the Office of the Director (Chapter 1).

OER (http://grants.nih.gov) is where you will find funding opportunity announcements (FOAs), application instructions, electronic research administration (eRA Commons), and all manner of grants and research-related policy statements. You will find tips and tutorials on preparing applications, on the review process, and on complying with NIH policy once you have an award. You will find a treasure trove of data on current and past awards and a variety of trends (Chapter 6). You will find detailed help specific to new and early stage investigators, training and career development, small business, and contracts. Their Web site is relatively well organized and easily navigated, so we will mainly address a few of their service areas in terms of how they can be integrated with your grant application strategy.

Funding Opportunities

Before you even begin to develop your research ideas, you first need to know what research the NIH wants to fund, particularly that sought by your IC(s) of interest. You are writing for the reviewers (Chapter 3) to conduct science that will advance progress toward achieving your IC's mission. Considering the FOAs available should be part of your proposal planning, and OER specifically offers advice on this strategy (http://grants.nih.gov/grants/planning_application.htm).

The Parent Announcements (http://grants.nih.gov/grants/guide/parent_announcements.htm) allow you to propose research on any topic of your choosing. This is also referred to as investigator-initiated research. Many ICs do not participate in the R21 and R03 parent announcements, however, and some have their own "parent" announcements for specific mechanisms (e.g., NCI has its own omnibus PAs for investigator-initiated R21 proposals). You will want to be sure your IC of choice participates in your parent announcement of choice.

Requests for Applications (RFAs) are FOAs with one or just a few atypical deadlines on a focused topic supported by a specific mechanism administered by one or more ICs. These are special initiatives that have been planned, approved by Council, and supported by funds set aside for this purpose. The RFA text will indicate the estimated number of awards to be made (and the budget limits for awarded applications, as applicable). In the Appendix, you can follow the "cleared concept" links to anticipate RFAs before they are published (Council approves or "clears" concepts, which the IC in turn converts into FOAs, often RFAs).

Program Announcements (PAs) allow ICs to indicate their interest in a specific area of research supported by a specific funding mechanism. Occasionally they set aside funds for these programs (PAS) or have specified receipt dates and review processes (PARs), but most follow the standard receipt dates (http://grants.nih.gov/grants/funding/submissionschedule.htm) and application format and are referred to CSR study sections for review (Chapter 3). OER explains the various FOAs in more detail (http://grants.nih.gov/grants/planning_application.htm#search).

New and updated FOAs are issued daily in the NIH Guide to Grants and Contracts (http://grants.nih.gov/grants/guide/index.html), which can be browsed (click on the column headings of the tables on the RFA, PA, and Notices pages to sort by that column) or searched. In addition, you can (and should) subscribe (http://grants.nih.gov/grants/guide/listserv.htm) to the weekly LISTSERV digest of all RFAs, Program Announcements (PAs, PARs, PASs), and Notices issued in the past week; Notices include new or changed grant policy, contract opportunities, requests for information (such as advance input on a planned research initiative), findings of research misconduct, alerts to upcoming FOAs, and any other announcements the NIH needs to make, so please take note of Notices as they are issued.

To subscribe, send an e-mail to listserv@list.nih.gov with the following text in the message body (not the Subject line):

subscribe NIHTOC-L your name
(e.g., subscribe NIHTOC-L Jeremy Berg)

Your address will be automatically obtained from the message.

Although subscribing to or regularly browsing the Guide will help you keep up with new opportunities and important policy announcements, generally you will want to know if there is a current FOA focused on a particular area of research or using a particular mechanism (e.g., if you want to repurpose an unfunded R01 as an R21 or as a new application to an appropriate RFA—more on what to do with unfunded applications in Chapter 13).

In the example shown in Figure 4.1 of a search for the term "personalized medicine," all types of FOAs are available for various mechanisms from different ICs. Often other ICs participate in funding announcements, so you should not assume an opportunity is not appropriate simply because your IC is not the issuing organization. For example, the first RFA is issued by the NIH Roadmap (Common Fund), which means it is a trans-NIH opportunity, but the second RFA, listed as issued by NIA, is likewise trans-NIH.

When reviewing an FOA, you will want to be sure that:

- an IC that is potentially interested in your science is participating,
- you are an eligible applicant, and
- there are no restrictions on the number of applications from your institution.

For some FOA, the applicant institution—that is, the university or perhaps each school within the university—can only submit one application, in which case you should inquire at your office of research or sponsored programs about the internal vetting process to select the single institutional applicant.

You will also want to review the scientific objectives to be sure what you want to do is what the IC wants to fund. If you are at all unsure whether your science is appropriate, ask the PO (Scientific/Research Contact) listed in the FOA. There is no use putting the time and effort into an application proposing research that is not appropriate for the program.

You will want to check the application receipt date for RFAs and PARs and the expiration date for all FOAs to ensure you can prepare your submission

Funding Opportunities & Notices Search Results
Active Funding Opportunities (RFAs & PAs)

Related Links:
- Funding Opportunities & Notices
- Advanced Funding Ops Search
- Advanced OER Site Search
- Search Help

Search Term(s): personalized medicine
Search within Results Below: [   ] (Search)

Matching Records: 13   Sorted by: Release Date (Desc) *

Announcement Number	Related Announc.	Issuing Organization	Release Date *	Opening Date (SF424 Only) ?	Expiration Date	Activity Code(s)	Title
RFA-RM-12-024	See Related	Roadmap	11/21/2012	01/28/2013	03/01/2013	U01	Determinants and Consequences of Personalized Health Care and Prevention (U01)
RFA-RM-12-023	See Related	NIA	11/16/2012	01/28/2013	03/01/2013	U01	Diffusion of Medical Technology and Effects on Outcomes and Expenditures (U01)
RFA-GM-14-001	See Related	NIGMS	10/17/2012	12/14/2012	01/16/2013	R01	Dynamics of Host-Associated Microbial Communities (R01)
PA-12-191	See Related	NIAMS	05/31/2012	11/05/2012	09/08/2015	R43, R44	Multiplex Assay Development for Arthritis and Musculoskeletal and Skin Diseases (SBIR [R43/R44])
PA-11-317	See Related	NIDCR	08/19/2011	09/05/2011	09/08/2014	R01	Building a Genetic and Genomic Knowledge Base in Dental, Oral, and Craniofacial Diseases and Disorders (R01)
PA-11-009	See Related	NIGMS	10/14/2010	01/12/2011	01/08/2014	K23	Translational Scholar Career Awards in Pharmacogenomics and Personalized Medicine (K23)
PAS-10-246	See Related	NIAAA	08/04/2010	09/05/2010	09/08/2013	R01	Strategies for Treatment of Young Adults with Alcohol Use Disorders (R01)
PAS-10-247	See Related	NIAAA	08/04/2010	09/16/2010	09/08/2013	R03	Strategies for Treatment of Young Adults with Alcohol Use Disorders (R03)
PAS-10-248	See Related	NIAAA	08/04/2010	09/16/2010	09/08/2013	R21	Strategies for Treatment of Young Adults with Alcohol Use Disorders (R21)
PAR-10-169	See Related	NCI	04/16/2010	05/05/2010	05/08/2013	R01	Academic-Industrial Partnerships for Translation of in vivo Imaging Systems for Cancer Investigations (R01)

FIGURE 4.1 The NIH Guide to Grants and Contracts (http://grants1.nih.gov/grants/guide/index.html) can be searched by keyword, here "personalized medicine," to identify FOAs appropriate for your research (OER has updated the appearance of the Guide, but the data are the same).

in time. PAs that are about to expire may be reissued, but you cannot count on this and should contact the PO listed in the FOA. You should also check to see whether a letter of intent (LOI) is requested (generally a month before the application receipt date). The LOI is for administrative purposes to help the PO and SRO anticipate the number and breadth of reviewers required and to identify any potential reviewers they had in mind who will be part of an application and hence unable to serve on the study section. The LOI is not required and only requests the proposed title and names of key personnel and participating institutions, not actual aims or an abstract—though you should discuss these separately with the PO when you start to develop the application, as discussed in Chapters 2 and 10.

The FOA will have the electronic application package embedded (click on the Apply for Grant Electronically button just above the Table of Contents), which you or your grants administrator must download to complete and submit via grants.gov; you will need to work with your individual institution, usually a sponsored programs or equivalent office, to learn how to submit the application, as this is specific to your institution.

The FOA will list any budget constraints or requirements and any additional instructions for preparing the application. You must read all the instructions for every FOA you consider. OER has streamlined these to eliminate much of the redundant administrative text, such that the key FOA-specific information and instructions are quickly and easily reviewed.

For FOAs that have multiple receipt dates or that have been reissued, you will want to search RePORTER to see what sort of projects submitted in response to the FOA have received awards, both to gauge what is of interest to the reviewers and ICs and to confirm that what you are about to propose has not already been funded.

For example, Figure 4.2 shows the results of a search for PA-11-009 from Figure 4.1. This FOA was issued in 2010 (FY11), and six awards had been made by 2013 (five by NIGMS and one by NICHD).

These data can help you decide whether the FOA is appropriate for what you want to propose. While you are here in RePORTER, clicking on the "Similar Projects" column icon will bring up a list of awards for similar research supported by all mechanisms and ICs (see Figure 4.3).

This is useful in gauging the extent to which your research focus may already be represented in your IC's portfolio. If they have funded similar studies, they may not be as enthusiastic about funding your work, so you would want to talk with the PO about tweaking your project to fill an important niche. You might also identify new POs at different ICs likely to have an interest in your research. In the example shown in Figure 4.3, please note that the fourth award down, 1ZIADK069075-15, is for intramural rather than extramural research, but you still do not want to duplicate this line of work; however, if your interests are complementary to those described in the intramural project, you might contact the PI to determine whether a collaboration might be possible since there are funding opportunities for intramural-extramural collaborative research (e.g., through the NIH Clinical Center http://www.cc.nih.gov/translational-research-resources/index.html, though basic science collaborations with intramural scientists can also be planned).

Project Search Results

Back to Query Form | Save Query | Share Query

Export All Projects GO

PROJECTS | PUBLICATIONS | PATENTS | CLINICAL STUDIES | DATA & VISUALIZE | MAP | LINKS | NEWS & MORE

There were 6 results matching your search criteria
Click on the column header to sort the results

Show/Hide Search Criteria

T: Application Type, Act: Activity Code, Project: Admin IC,Serial No., Year: Support Year/Supplement/Amendment

T	Act	Project	Year	Sub #	Project Title	Contact PI/ Project Leader	Organization	FY	Admin IC	Funding IC	FY Total Cost by IC	Similar Projects
5	K23	GM100183	02		PHARMACOGENOMICS OF TACROLIMUS AND NEW ONSET DIABETES AFTER KIDNEY TRANSPLANT	BIRDWELL, KELLY A	VANDERBILT UNIVERSITY MED CTR	2012	NIGMS	NCATS	$188,460	
5	K23	GM100273	02		ADIPONECTIN POLYMORPHISMS, INSULIN RESISTANCE, AND PHARMACOKINETICS IN OBESITY	INGRANDE, JERRY	STANFORD UNIVERSITY	2012	NIGMS	NCATS	$196,288	
5	K23	GM100372	02		STATIN PHARMACOGENOMICS: A MULTI-GENE PK-PD MODELING APPROACH	KITZMILLER, JOSEPH PAUL	OHIO STATE UNIVERSITY	2012	NIGMS	NCATS	$191,052	
1	K23	GM102678	01		ASPIRIN PHARMACOGENOMICS: ROLE OF PEAR1 IN PERSONALIZED ANTI-PLATELET THERAPY	LEWIS, JOSHUA PATRICK	UNIVERSITY OF MARYLAND BALTIMORE	2012	NIGMS	NIGMS	$161,218	
1	K23	HD000001	01		MTRNR1 AMINOGLYCOSIDE OTOTOXICITY OUTCOMES AND PARENTAL PERCEPTIONS OF TESTING	MCGREGOR, TRACY L.	VANDERBILT UNIVERSITY MED CTR	2012	NICHD	NICHD	$175,920	
1	K23	GM100288	01A1		THE 1200 PATIENTS PROJECT: STUDYING CLINICAL IMPLEMENTATION OF PHARMACOGENOMICS	O'DONNELL, PETER HUGH	UNIVERSITY OF CHICAGO	2013	NIGMS	NIGMS	$189,648	

FIGURE 4.2 RePORTER (http://projectreporter.nih.gov/reporter.cfm) can be searched by FOA to identify which applications submitted in response to your targeted FOA have received funding. Note the final column with a button linking to "Similar Projects."

Project Number: 5K23GM100273-02
Title: ADIPONECTIN POLYMORPHISMS, INSULIN RESISTANCE, AND PHARMACOKINETICS IN OBESITY
Contact PI / Project Leader: INGRANDE, JERRY
Awardee Organization: STANFORD UNIVERSITY

100 projects similar to 5K23GM100273-02 (100 maximum).
Modify List of Similar Projects
Click on the column header to sort the results
Records per page 25
Page 1 of 4 Next Last

Match Score	Project Number	Sub #	Project Title	Contact PI / Project Leader	Organization	FY	Admin IC	Funding IC	FY Total Cost by IC
531	5R01HD040787-13		STUDY TO INVESTIGATE THE PATHOPHYSIOLOGY OF TYPE 2 DIABETES IN YOUTH	CAPRIO, SONIA	YALE UNIVERSITY	2012	NICHD	NICHD	$366,010
530	5R01DK078112-04		ADIPOKINES IN HEMODIALYSIS PATIENTS	BEDDHU, SRINIVASAN	UNIVERSITY OF UTAH	2011	NIDDK	NIDDK	$553,439
526	5R01DK080743-05		LIPOCALIN 2 IN INFLAMMATION AND METABOLIC CONTROL	CHEN, XIAOLI	UNIVERSITY OF MINNESOTA TWIN CITIES	2012	NIDDK	NIDDK	$284,014
523	1ZIADK069075-15		GENE EXPRESSION PROFILING ON INSULIN RESISTANCE AND OBESITY	BOGARDUS, CLIFTON	NATIONAL INSTITUTE OF DIABETES AND DIGESTIVE AND KIDNEY DISEASES	2012	NIDDK	NIDDK	$1,088,344
520	5P01HL081587-07	7342	ADIPOSE TISSUE INFLAMMATION & VASCULARITY	WALSH, KENNETH	BOSTON UNIVERSITY MEDICAL CAMPUS	2012	NHLBI		$532,415
506	5R01DK084171-03		CTRP9, A NOVEL ADIPOSE TISSUE-SECRETED GLYCOPROTEIN	WONG, GUANG WILLIAM	JOHNS HOPKINS UNIVERSITY	2012	NIDDK	NIDDK	$340,144
504	5U54HD012303-32	6875	PROJECT 2 - METABOLIC CONTROL OF REPRODUCTION	OLEFSKY, JERROLD MICHAEL	UNIVERSITY OF CALIFORNIA AT SAN DIEGO	2012	NICHD		$386,471
491	5K23HL092069-03		CHANGES IN ADIPOKINES AND ADIPOSITY DURING PUBERTY AND YOUNG ADULTHOOD	MIHALOPOULOS, NICOLE LENORE	UNIVERSITY OF UTAH	2012	NHLBI	NHLBI	$142,560

FIGURE 4.3 RePORTER (http://projectreporter.nih.gov/reporter.cfm) returned this list of funded applications upon clicking on the Similar Projects link for award number 5K32GM100273-02 (see Figure 4.2).

Preparing Your Application

Once you have identified an appropriate FOA, you will also want to download the application package instructions for the SF424 (http://grants.nih.gov/grants/forms.htm). OER has other forms and instructions available for specific application and reporting uses, but most PIs will only need to understand the SF424 package. The main point to remember here is to confirm that you have the most recent version whenever you are preparing an application and need to check the instructions for a particular detail. Most PIs ignore the SF424 instructions, but you will find useful information and should especially focus on the instructions for Completing PHS 398 Components.

OER, like many ICs, offers guidance and tutorials on the application and review process for new and established investigators alike, which we list here but will not go through:

- Planning Your Application (http://grants.nih.gov/grants/planning_application.htm)
- Types of Funding Mechanisms (http://grants.nih.gov/grants/funding/funding_program.htm)
- How to Apply (http://grants.nih.gov/grants/how_to_apply.htm)
- Writing Your Application (http://grants.nih.gov/grants/writing_application.htm)
- Submitting Your Application (http://grants.nih.gov/grants/submitapplication.htm)
- Applying Electronically (http://grants.nih.gov/grants/ElectronicReceipt/index.htm)
- Peer Review Process (http://grants.nih.gov/grants/peer_review_process.htm)
- NIH Regional Grant Seminars on Program Funding and Grants Administration (http://grants.nih.gov/grants/seminars.htm)

While most of these are self-explanatory, you will definitely want to explore the Regional Grants Seminar page, both to keep alert to register for the next seminar (quite valuable to attend, especially for those new to the grant application process) and to review the individual PowerPoint presentations made available by some host sites (e.g., OHSU/Portland, Oregon in June 2010, http://www.ohsu.edu/xd/research/nih-regional-seminar.cfm). These seminars cover every aspect of the grant application and review process, working with NIH personnel, postaward management, and many specialized and late-breaking topics, and offer hands-on computer training for the eRA Commons. OER also organizes workshops (http://grants.nih.gov/grants/ outreach.htm) on SBIR/STTR programs and animal welfare.

eRA Commons

Although you will work directly with your PO and your IC-assigned Grant Management Specialist (GMS) on the postaward management of your grant, OER does maintain the interface through which all application-related inter-action with the NIH occurs: the NIH eRA Commons. You will go here to track the status of your applications as they are submitted through grants. gov, assigned for review, discussed (or not) by study sections, considered by Council for funding, and selected (or not) for an award. You will be able to review the application package, the referral receipt, and summary statement as these documents become available. You will submit Just-in-Time (JIT) information through the eRA Commons link for that application. The eRA Commons screen shot in Figure 4.4 displays the management of an awarded application, which includes the history from submission through all Notices of Award (new and noncompeting renewals).

If you receive an award, you will conduct all postaward management (progress reports, financial reports, no-cost extensions, closeout) through the Commons, including the management of training and career development awards (via xTrain, http://era.nih.gov/training_career/index.cfm). You can also access My NCBI to track your grant-related publications in accordance with the NIH Public Access Policy (http://publicaccess.nih.gov), which is being strictly enforced, such that your noncompeting renewal will be held up if you are in noncompliance (Chapter 14).

If you serve as a reviewer, eRA Commons will be your portal for signing conflict of interest forms, accessing applications, and posting scores and cri-tiques as part of the Internet-Assisted Review (IAR) process. Some reviews are conducted online as well (Chapter 3).

If you do not already have an eRA Commons User Name and account, you will ask your current institution (generally the sponsored programs or research office) to set one up for you. This is a lifetime account that will fol-low you wherever you move in the course of your career. When selecting your eRA Commons User Name, keep in mind this is for keeps and should allow others to identify you (i.e., do not be creative or use an online dating site-type handle). You will be required to change your password regularly, so this is definitely not a one-time decision.

General Grant Information

Status:	Application awarded
Institution Name:	UNIVERSITY OF PITTSBURGH AT PITTSBURGH
School Name:	SCHOOL OF MEDICINE
School Category:	SCHOOLS OF MEDICINE
Division Name:	NONE
Department Name:	MEDICINE
PI Name:	WHITCOMB, DAVID C
Application ID:	1R01DK077906-01A2
Proposal Title:	NAPS2-AS: Race Dependent Risk for Pancreatitis
Proposal Receipt Date:	03/09/2009
Last Status Update Date:	05/06/2010
Current Award Notice Date:	03/15/2011
Application Source:	Grants.gov
Project Period Begin Date:	05/15/2010
Project Period End Date:	03/31/2014
eApplication Status:	Submission Complete
FOA:	[PA07-070] - RESEARCH PROJECT GRANT (PARENT R01)
NIH Appl. ID:	7785736

Other Relevant Documents

- e-Application
- Appendix: Archives manuscript accepted version
- Appendix 2: Fum v1.0-021809
- Appendix 3: Fup v1.0-021809
- appendix 4: Naps2 code book may 08
- Appendix 5: Edcguide2008
- Summary Statement
- latest NGA
- Notice(s) of Grant Award (PDF): 03/15/2011 12/14/2010 05/11/2010
- Abstract (Awarded Grant)
- Just in Time: 09/07/2009 Times Revised(1)
- Submission Cover Letter
- Notifications for Review (0 documents)

Correspondence

Referral		
Date	Description	Action

Status History

Effective Date	Status Message
05/06/2010	Award prepared: refer questions to Grants Management Specialist.
03/05/2010	Pending administrative review. Refer any questions to Program Official or Grants Management Specialist.
09/10/2009	Council review completed.
07/22/2009	Scientific Review Group review completed: Council review pending. Refer any questions to Program Official.
03/17/2009	Scientific Review Group review pending. Refer any questions to the Scientific Review Administrator.
03/09/2009	Application entered into system

Institute or Center Assignment

Institute or Center	Assignment Date
NATIONAL INSTITUTE OF ALLERGY AND INFECTIOUS DISEASES	03/12/2009
NATIONAL INSTITUTE OF DIABETES AND DIGESTIVE AND KIDNEY DISEASES (Primary)	03/09/2009
NATIONAL INSTITUTE OF DIABETES AND DIGESTIVE AND KIDNEY DISEASES (Primary)	03/12/2009
NATIONAL INSTITUTE ON ALCOHOL ABUSE AND ALCOHOLISM	03/12/2009

Application Information

Award Document Number:	RDK077906A
FSR Accepted Code:	N
Snap Indicator Code:	Y
Impact Score:	22
Percentile:	10.0
Early Stage Investigator Eligible:	N
New Investigator Eligible:	N
Eligible for FFATA Reporting:	No

Study Section

Scientific Review Group:	ZDK1 GRB-R (O2)
Council Meeting Date(YYYY/MM):	2009/10
Meeting Date:	07/22/2009
Meeting Time:	04:00
Study Roster:	View Meeting Roster

Advisory Council(AC) Information

Meeting Date:	09/09/2009
Meeting Time:	08:30

FIGURE 4-4 You will monitor the status of your submitted applications and manage your funded applications, such as the example shown here, through your eRA Commons account (https://public.era.nih.gov/commons/public/login.do). Notice that the application, summary statement, Just-in-Time (JIT), Notices of (Grant) Award (NGA) for each fiscal year, and other documents are all accessible here.

The eRA Commons Web site (http://era.nih.gov/applicants/index.cfm) includes a Demo site to practice using eRA Commons features, step-by-step instructions, and a very responsive help desk. Once you have submitted an application, you will likely monitor its progress obsessively (phenotype applies to both new and established PIs). Please note that delays in updates to you eRA Commons status are not unusual and are generally not worrisome and that communication with your PO will be a better gauge of what is happening with your application. However, please also note that your application status will only change to reflect an award that is to be or has been made. Your eRA Commons status will not reflect the fact that your application is no longer under consideration for funding; the status will remain stuck at "Council review completed" until the application is administratively withdrawn years later.

Grants Policy

As we noted at the outset, OER manages all grants policy at the agency level. New and updates to current policy are announced as Notices in the NIH Guide, and you should keep alert to these, which are also listed on the OER grants policy page (http://grants.nih.gov/grants/policy/policy.htm). The NIH Nexus (http://nexus.od.nih.gov/all/) and OER blog (http://nexus.od.nih.gov/all/rock-talk/) cover policy issues, especially new and modified policy components, in detail. The Rock Talk blog is also responsive to comments posted by the extramural community. One example of a policy change and its subsequent re-evaluation is the decision not to accept a second amended application (A2), which OER reviewed with data (http://nexus.od.nih.gov/all/2012/11/28/the-a2-resubmission-policy-continues-a-closer-look-at-recent-data/).

You as an NIH applicant or grantee will want to bookmark the NIH Grants Policy Statement (http://grants.nih.gov/grants/policy/policy.htm), which can be browsed via the hyperlinked table of contents or searched. Your grants administrator should know this inside and out, but you should keep familiar with policies that affect your grant strategy.

In addition to application submission and award management, the major areas of grants and research policy overseen by OER include the following:

- NIH Public Access: http://publicaccess.nih.gov
- Peer Review Policies and Practices: http://grants.nih.gov/grants/peer/peer.htm

- Compliance and Oversight (mainly institutional but also the NIH financial conflict of interest policy, which is relevant to every applicant and awardee): http://grants.nih.gov/grants/compliance/compliance.htm
- Research Involving Human Subjects: http://grants.nih.gov/grants/policy/hs/index.htm
- Animals in Research: http://grants.nih.gov/grants/policy/air/index.htm and http://grants.nih.gov/grants/olaw/olaw.htm (Office of Laboratory Animal Welfare)
- Intellectual Property Policy: http://grants.nih.gov/grants/intell-property.htm and https://s-edison.info.nih.gov/iEdison/ (invention reporting)
- Research Integrity: http://grants.nih.gov/grants/research_integrity/index.htm

With regard to the last item, Research Integrity, you should be aware that an office outside the NIH, the Office of Research Integrity (ORI, http://www.ori.dhhs.gov), is responsible for investigation allegations of research misconduct. ORI is not part of the NIH because this office must be independent and able to investigate intramural researchers at the NIH as well as investigators funded by other agencies in the Department of Health and Human Services (HHS). Their findings of misconduct are published in the Federal Register and as Notices in the NIH Guide to Grants and Contracts (if NIH funding is involved). ORI has many excellent resources for responsible conduct of research (RCR) training, such as an interactive role-playing video with branching outcomes depending on the decisions made along the way; The Lab: Avoiding Research Misconduct (http://ori.hhs.gov/thelab) is available in English, Spanish and Chinese, and ORI is currently working on another interactive video tool to address research misconduct in the clinical setting.

Finally, the NIH has policies specific to new investigators (that is, those who have never received a substantial NIH independent research award regardless of their seniority) and early stage investigators (ESI) (those who are new investigators within 10 years of their terminal research degree or medical residency). The ESI designation was added to distinguish investigators near the beginning of their independent careers from senior researchers competing for their first NIH award (e.g., established NIH intramural or foreign researchers who relocated to an American university or research institution). These policies are designed to help these junior applicants compete with established investigators and secure independent support earlier than the current average age of 42 for those with a PhD and 44 or older for those with an MD. The New and Early Stage Investigator Policies Web site (http://grants1.nih.gov/grants/new_investigators/index.htm) provides the latest information on the definition of new investigator and ESI applicants, policy updates, links to IC-specific policies and practices, employment and success rates, and current funding opportunities targeting this cohort of researchers. For the Pathway to Independence (K99-R00) program in particular, applicants and awardees will want to be in close communication with their PO, since each IC manages this mechanism somewhat differently (http://grants1.nih.gov/grants/guide/contacts/parent_K99_R00.html).

5

Federal Budget Process

IF YOUR APPLICATION is discussed, as soon as you get the overall impact score, your first question will inevitably be, is this good enough to be funded? The answer to this question depends, of course, on the score/percentile itself... and on the time of year.

Principal investigators (PIs) often do not appreciate the degree to which the federal budget process dictates NIH grant-making activities. Unless you have a score of 10 or are in the 1st to 5th percentile, your Program Officer (PO) may truly not know whether you will be considered for funding since your Institute or Center (IC) may not know about its funding from Congress. In 2013, for example, a series of "fiscal cliffs" delayed the federal budget until the fiscal year was more than half over, such that most awards were not made until April or May (or later), and then at very conservative levels due to the budget cut imposed by sequestration. Table 1.1 in Chapter 1 lays out a timeline illustrating Congressional budget activities in parallel with IC grant-making decisions, though here we will describe the process in detail.

Officially, the federal fiscal year (FY) starts on October 1, with the subsequent calendar year assigned (e.g., FY14 started October 1, 2013). However, it has been more than a decade since Congress has approved appropriation bills for the various federal agencies, including the NIH, in time for the start of an fiscal year. This means that each IC has little clarity about how much money it will have for the fiscal year and therefore can not plan meaningfully. This is no way to run a railroad or build the national biomedical research enterprise, but this is the dysfunctional system we have.

NIH planning for each fiscal year starts more than a full year in advance. In the spring, the Office of the Director of the NIH requests information from the ICs and uses this information to develop an overall budget for NIH that is transmitted to the Department of Health and Human Services (HHS). Based on this input, HHS forwards its agency-wide proposed plan to the Office of Management and Budget (OMB), usually in October, shortly after the start of the fiscal year preceding the one for which the budget is being planned (i.e., in October 2013 for FY14). OMB examines this budget proposal and sends a revised budget (referred to as the "passback budget") to the agencies, usually over the winter holiday break. The NIH can then appeal this budget, first to HHS and, if HHS agrees, to OMB. Decisions are made based on these appeals, leading to the President's Budget, a financial proposal for the entire federal government for the upcoming fiscal year, which is released to Congress and the public, usually on the first Monday in February. Exceptions to this time line do occur, as for FY14, when the plan was not submitted to Congress until April 2013.

Whether Congress treats this document as the framework for the next fiscal year budget depends on which party is in the White House and which parties are in charge of the houses of Congress. The appropriation bills introduced for each federal agency may or may not bear any resemblance to the President's request. Often the budget proposal for the NIH is conservative to enhance the likelihood that it will be accepted—and possibly increased—by Congress (and hence an amount the NIH can feel somewhat confident on planning for).

The Congressional Budget Office completes its analysis of the President's plan by March. Like the President, the House and Senate prepare their own budget resolutions (usually by mid-April) that broadly outline spending categories, targets, revenues, and spending estimates (outlays) for the next fiscal year. This guides the Appropriations Committees and Subcommittees as they set funding levels for federal agencies.

The Director of the NIH and, often, the directors of some ICs testify at appropriate House and Senate Committee and Subcommittee (see Chapter 1) hearings on behalf of their budget requests and provide updates on specific programs, particularly those cited in prior appropriation bills. Generally, this occurs in the spring (March-April).

Groups outside the government work behind the scenes with Subcommittee staff to optimize the appropriation for their agency of interest (e.g., many patient advocacy groups lobby on behalf of the NIH). The Federation of American Societies for Experimental Biology (FASEB) manages a program that brings scientists to Washington for just this purpose and makes available a Congressional Visit Toolbox for anyone who might be interested in advocating for NIH funding (http://www.faseb.org/Policy-and-Government-Affairs/Advocacy-on-Capitol-Hill/Congressional-Visit-Toolbox.aspx). Many scientific societies also engage Congress prior to the passage of appropriation bills, so be sure to check with those with which you are affiliated. Subcommittee chairs have considerable influence in drafting appropriation bills, so it is important to target their staff in addition to elected delegations from your state and district.

Full Committees on Appropriations review Subcommittee reports before drafting the 12 appropriations bills for their respective houses of Congress. Enacted appropriations bills all originate in the House (per the Constitution), but the Senate passes their own and later concurs, generally with amendments, with the House version. Although the timing varies significantly, and some reports never even get out of Committee, you can check the progress and substance of the NIH appropriation at Thomas (http://thomas.loc.gov/home/thomas.php); click on the Appropriations Bills link and look for the "Labor/HHS/Education" row.

Members of the House and Senate then debate, amend, and vote on their respective appropriation bills, which is often the only time most legislators get to voice their opinions, since Congressional leaders in each house carefully control the size and membership of Committees. A joint Conference Committee reconciles the two bills (another opportunity for lobbying on behalf of specific budget items), and both chambers vote on the final bill. Often, due to repeated delays and disagreements, the multiple appropriations are distilled into a single "omnibus" bill for the entire federal government months after the October 1 start of the fiscal year.

The President then signs the bill into law (a veto is very unlikely at this point), and the ICs allocate their appropriations, taking into consideration any restrictions, specified funding requirements, or other directed language in the enacted law (more on this later).

If Congress fails to pass appropriation bills by October 1, they must pass a Continuing Resolution (CR) to fund the federal government, usually continuing the same funding level of the previous fiscal year, though CRs have been proposed (but not passed) that are based on much earlier fiscal years, such that the CR would represent a significant budget cut. The CR legislation is enacted for a specified period, with additional CRs passed as needed to keep the government operation—sometimes for months, sometimes essentially for the entire year (as in FY07, FY11, and FY13).

These delays are awkward for the ICs because IC staff do not know how much money they will have available and whether their appropriation might in fact drop when a budget bill is finally enacted, as occurred following sequestration in FY13. This uncertainty also delays the funding of many grants and programs. While under a CR, the ICs can make only a limited number of new grant awards (those with the best scores or the highest programmatic priority) and fund ongoing awards at a reduced level than was originally approved. The ICs are also prohibited by law from launching new initiatives outside the scope of the existing authorization while a CR is in effect.

This entire process starts from scratch every year, with the current fiscal year budget being executed and two subsequent fiscal year budgets in different stages of development.

Once the President has signed an appropriations or omnibus bill into law, the Office of Management and Budget makes funds available to HHS, which makes funds available to the NIH, which makes funds available to each IC. Only at this point, when the ICs know their final funding level for the fiscal year, can they determine the number of awards they can make and hence estimate their paylines or paylists (Chapter 2). The National Cancer Institute has summarized the calculation process like this:

Step 1: From the amount appropriated by Congress, deduct:
- The amount of noncompeting commitments, including the cost of program evaluation
- The amount for mandated set-asides (e.g., SBIR)
- The amount for program initiatives (RFAs)
  This leaves the amount for competing grants.
Step 2: From the amount remaining for competing grants (generally ~20% of the appropriation):
- Distribute to the main mechanisms (R01, P01) and the smaller mechanisms (R03, R21, R33)
- Hold approximately 5%–10% in reserve for select pay/exceptions
- Distribute the exception reserve to Program Division Director for supplements and exceptions
- Allocate across each of the three review rounds
Step 3: Based on historical data and current review results, set paylines for research project grants (RPGs).

Thus, even once the law establishing the budget for the fiscal year is signed, it takes several weeks for each IC to sort out its funding range, so you should not expect an answer about an application that may have been in limbo for months immediately after a federal budget is passed. You must remember, too, as just outlined, that most of each IC's appropriation is already committed to ongoing grants and that, depending on the timing of the final budget, the ICs may need to wait for all grant applications to be reviewed before they can estimate their final funding range for applications reviewed earlier.

This is why those ICs that do publish interim paylines (e.g., NIAID, NHLBI, NIAMS) start with very conservative percentiles and scores; if the payline is raised later in the fiscal year, which it usually is (but not always), applications from earlier cycles that also fall within the higher payline will be picked up later for funding. Toward the end of the fiscal year (around August), the ICs calculate how much money they have remaining to fund applications nominated (by POs) for select pay (that is, funded above the payline). ICs want to avoid having to lower their final paylines from interim levels, though this has happened (e.g., National Institute of Environmental Health Sciences in FY13).

Although the NIH tries to plan budgets on 3-year cycles (see Table 1.1 in Chapter 1), each fiscal year is managed individually, and ICs can no longer even count on future appropriations to keep pace with inflation, much less support new major initiatives. Currently, the NIH is authorized by Congress to maintain an average award length of 4 years, with shorter awards offsetting those approved for 5 years of funding. However, with the recent focus on debt and deficit reduction, ICs may be working more diligently to shorten the duration of all awards, so they are not caught with too large of a long-term commitment should a severe budget cut be imposed again, as with sequestration in FY13. Therefore, part of your application planning strategy should include discussion with your PO of project—and therefore budget—size and duration (e.g., fewer aims, shorter project period, smaller budget).

At the conclusion of the fiscal year, each IC is busy making final awards, closing out their books, and preparing progress reports from the current fiscal year to accompany budget requests for the next fiscal year. In general, no carryover of funds by the IC is allowed by law (though PIs can carry funds over, as discussed in Chapter 14), so that the ICs strive to conclude the fiscal year with a zero balance. Once the next fiscal year begins, competing grants are not paid, fellowships are not activated, and awards are not transferred from one institution to another until mid- to late November at the earliest, usually closer to December 1 to be in line with major NIH funding cycles. You can monitor when "your" IC starts making awards via the *Notice of Grant Awards issued within the last 90 days* Excel file on the NIH Budget and Spending Web site, http://report.nih.gov/budget_and_spending/index.aspx). Even if you have been told that your Cycle 1 application (February–March submission) with a score of 10 will be funded, you should not expect activity on this until later in November. Your institution could set up an account for approved research charges up to 90 days before the Notice of Award is issued, but you will need to work this out with your sponsored programs or comparable office and your department (all of whom will want confirmation from your PO or Grants Management Specialist that an award will be issued and at what level—almost certainly not at your requested total costs).

6

NIH Funding Data and Trends

AS A SCIENTIST, you do not need to be convinced of the importance of obtaining and analyzing the best possible data. Planning and preparing competitive applications will involve more than data from your scientific investigations. Although in some cases, you will have no choice about the funding opportunity, mechanism, or Institute or Center (IC) to target, often you will have different options, both in the short term and as part of a long-term grant application strategy. Your Program Officer (PO) will be able to answer many questions specific to his or her IC, but at times, you will want to look at the bigger picture to observe funding trends over time and by applicant cohort (that is, your peers specifically).

The Office of Extramural Research (Chapter 4) maintains NIH-wide data on applications, applicants, and review and award trends. The manner in which they present these data to the extramural community has been expanded and refined significantly over the years, such that it is relatively easy (and sometimes even a pleasure) to track down much of what you need. In fact, if you have a specific question, you can ask it, including via smartphone voice recognition interface, in plain language through the Funding Facts page (http://report.nih.gov/fundingfacts/index.cfm). NIH Deputy Director for Extramural Research Sally Rockey walks you through how to use these features on her blog (http://nexus.od.nih.gov/all/2012/10/05/report-funding-facts-why-don't-you-just-tell-us-what-you-want-to-know/), but as you can see in Figure 6.1, it is quite intuitive.

While Funding Facts is a good place to start with a quick question, the NIH Data Book (http://report.nih.gov/nihdatabook/index.aspx) is the compendium of all extramural research data. You can learn about the NIH

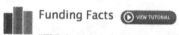 Funding Facts ⊙ VIEW TUTORIAL   FROZEN

NOTE: The figures in Funding Facts may differ from information appearing in official NIH Office of Budget and Institute/Center (IC) budget mechanism tables. In Funding Facts, the cost of each award is attributed to the IC administering the grant or contract even though funding for the award may have been provided by the NIH Office of the Director, another IC, or another source. Also, funding provided by the American Recovery and Reinvestment Act of 2009 is not included. For official budget information, see the NIH Office of Budget website at officeofbudget.od.nih.gov or individual IC websites. To use this tool, please make sure your browser's pop-up blocker is disabled.

What would you like to know?

[   ] ?

Query examples:
What was NIGMS's R01 success rate in 2011?
Funding for new R01s in 2011?
HL RPG awards?

[SUBMIT QUERY] [RESET QUERY]

Didn't find what you were looking for? Try Advanced Search.

ADVANCED SEARCH

Topic:	All	SELECT
Admin Institute/Center:	All NIH	SELECT
Funding Mechanism:	All	SELECT
Activity:	All in aggregate	SELECT
Type:	All Types in aggregate	SELECT
Fiscal Year:	2012	SELECT

[SUBMIT QUERY] [RESET QUERY]

FIGURE 6.1 Funding Facts can be searched via plain-language queries (http://report. nih.gov/fundingfacts/fundingfacts.aspx)

budget over the years, detailed demographic data on applicants (faculty, post-doc, student), and all success and funding rates (see Fig. 6.2).

In Chapter 2, we showed you FY12 R01 application funding trend data for some ICs, in terms of the number of applications reviewed and funded at each percentile (as high up as the individual IC went). In Table 6.1, we summarize the R01-equivalent (R01, R37, DP2) success rates for the entire NIH by application type and submission for FY03 and FY12 (Table 210 at http://report.nih.gov/success_rates/index.aspx). Note the increase in the number of new applications (keep in mind, too, that A2 applications could be submitted in FY03, whereas the FY12 numbers only reflect A1 submission, and the DP2 mechanism was not available in FY03) and declining number of awards in all categories.

As you can see, success rates have dropped in all categories in recent years. This table also highlights the better success rate of competing renewal (Type 2) R01s compared with new (Type 1) R01 applications: they both are scored and percentiled in the same study section and are held to the same pay-line, but the initial (A0) submission of a competing renewal is more than four times more likely to be funded than a new application. This is one reason why ICs prefer that their new and early stage investigator (ESI) applicants pursue R01s, since this mechanism can be renewed (unlike the R21 or R03), which is a less daunting task, assuming you have been productive in the prior fund-ing period. Now, this last point is critical to keep in mind as well; that is, the Type 2 applicant pool starts off much smaller and is even more self-selected, in that only those principal investigators (PIs) who have been productive and published during the last budget period will attempt to submit a competing renewal. Nonetheless, the renewable R01 remains the best route to securing a stable, independent career in biomedical research.

Table 6.1 NIH-wide success rate for R01-equivalent applications by application type and amendment status for FY03 and FY12

Application		FY03	FY12
Type	Submission		
1 (new)	A0	17.0% 13,539 applications, 2,303 awards	8.6% 19,259 applications, 1,662 awards
	A1+	42.8% 5,199 applications, 2,223 awards	37.2% 5,380 applications, 2,002 awards
2 (competing renewal)	A0	45.0% 3,922 applications, 1,765 awards	28.4% 3,201 applications, 910 awards
	A1+	58.7% 1,863 applications, 1,093 awards	49.7% 1,689 applications, 839 awards
3 (supplement)		41.4% 111 applications, 46 awards	24.5% 98 applications, 24 awards
Overall		30.2% 24,634 applications, 7,430 awards	18.4% 29,627 applications, 5,437 awards

Getting back to the available data resources, the Budget and Spending page (http://report.nih.gov/budget_and_spending/index.aspx) offers data on all aspects of the NIH budget and funding, including awards issued in the past 90 days (http://silk.nih.gov/public/cbz2z0z.@www.recent.awards.csv). This Excel spreadsheet is particularly useful if you are wondering whether your IC is making any new awards during times of budget uncertainty, such as throughout a continuing resolution (see Chapter 5).

Another interesting resource here is "Ways of Managing NIH Resources," which takes you to a modifiable presentation inviting comment on how best to manage the increasingly stressed NIH budget (http://report.nih.gov/budget_and_spending/index.aspx). You can see the impact of various tweaks by limiting award size, number of awards, or dollar amount to one PI, and PI salary (percent effort covered by NIH funds) (see Figure 6.3).

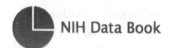

The NIH Data Book (NDB) provides basic summary statistics on extramural grants and contract awards, grant applications, the organizations that NIH supports, the trainees and fellows supported through NIH programs, and the national biomedical workforce. Tables and charts are provided in a variety of formats, including PowerPoint (PPT) slides and Portable Documents Files (PDF) files.

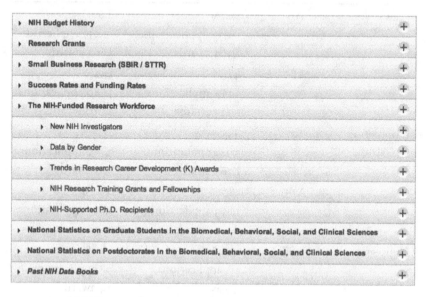

FIGURE 6.2 NIH Data Book presents a wide range of analyses (http://report.nih.gov/nihdatabook/index.aspx)

Depending on what you need to know for planning and strategy purposes, you can look at the number of applications and awards and success rate by almost any metric for the last decade: funding mechanism, IC, type of application (new, renewal, supplement), submission number (A0, A1), and various details about the applicant (http://report.nih.gov/success_rates/index.aspx). By clicking on the column headings for these Excel spreadsheets, you can customize the data presented to include specific ICs, FYs, activity codes, and other options. You can compare awards by location (applicant institution, department, etc.), if you want to take this into consideration as part of a job search or when comparing offers.

You can also check the level of support by area of research, disease, or condition (http://report.nih.gov/categorical_spending.aspx); in Figure 6.4, we show you the options starting with "A" to illustrate the diversity of categories (e.g., Agent Orange and Dioxin, Arctic, Assistive Technology, Asthma, etc.). These categories demonstrate the importance of the terms in your Project

Budget and Spending

<u>Ways of Managing NIH Resources</u>

<u>Funding Facts</u>

<u>NIH Office of Budget</u>

<u>Current Operating Year Budget</u>

<u>Summary of the President's Budget Request for NIH</u>

<u>NIH Online Performance Appendix</u>

Research Grants and Contracts

Notice of Grant Awards issued within the last 90 days	(~8MB)
Grants and Contracts: Number of awards and total funding, by budget mechanism and Institute/Center	(~160KB)

Research Grants

Research grants: Awards and total funding, by mechanism, type, and activity	(~154KB)
Research grants: Awards and total funding, by type and Institute/Center	(~62KB)
Research grants: Awards and total funding, by mechanism and activity	(~60KB)
Research grants: Total funding, current and constant dollars	(~51KB)
NIH Data Book: Research Grants	

FIGURE 6.3 Budget and Spending offers customizable spreadsheets of funding trend data (http://report.nih.gov/budget_and_spending/index.aspx)

RePORTER listing, though the NIH uses sophisticated data mining techniques to categorize and cluster terms and phrases for this database. Please note that the amounts reflect trends in NIH-wide funding associated with the term rather funds expressly budgeted for each disease area.

Applying Data to Your Application Strategy

You might not be so interested in the general funding trends, beyond the payline for your target IC(s), but these data can be useful in planning your overall application strategy. Table 6.2 shows the sort of data comparison a postdoc conducting basic cancer research (e.g., DNA repair following exposure to ultraviolet radiation) might put together when considering what mechanism (Chapter 7) and Institute (Chapter 2) to target. As we noted earlier, we have included the FY03 data for comparison with funding a decade ago, though if you were doing such an analysis, you would want to compare data for the two to three most fiscal years for which data are available (data from Tables 203, 204, and 206 at http://report.nih.gov/success_rates/index.aspx).

Table 6.2 Sample analysis by a postdoc engaged in DNA repair research to evaluate which funding mechanisms and ICs to target

Institute	Mechanism	FY03 Success Rate (applications/ awards)	FY12 Success Rate (applications/ awards)
National Cancer Institute	R01	21.3% (2,987/636)	12.5% (4,056/509)
	R03	43.3% (247/107)	20.0% (506/101)
	R15	40.0% (50/20)	9.7% (155/15)
	R21	22.7% (963/219)	9.8% (2,322/228)
	F32	21.5% (219/47)	18.1% (232/42)
	K01	32.1% (109/35)	55.6% (27/15)
	K22	26.7% (45/12)	14.6% (41/6)
	K99	NA	17.0% (147/25)
	Appropriation	$4.59B	$5.07B
National Institute of Environmental Health Sciences	R01	13.9% (274/38)	16.9% (444/75)
	R03	100% (1/1)	12.1% (58/7)
	R15	36.8% (19/7)	18.6% (43/8)
	R21	NA	10.4% (568/59)
	F32	53.3% (30/16)	26.5% (34/9)
	K01	0% (1/0)	50% (2/1)
	K22	26.3% (19/5)	NA
	K99	NA	38.1% (21/8)
	Appropriation	$698M	$764M
National Institute of General Medical Sciences	R01	25.4% (1,697/431)	18.2% (2,418/441)
	R03	100% (1/1)	NA
	R15	53.9% (89/48)	16.7% (282/47)
	R21	18.3% (71/13)	14.7% (170/25)
	F32	38.9% (460/179)	30.4% (504/153)
	K01	NA	NA
	K22	NA	NA
	K99	NA	13.0% (115/15)
	Appropriation	$1.84B	$2.43B

A few caveats. NIEHS is the only IC in this group that participates in the R03 and R21 parent announcements (NCI and NIGMS only accept applications for these activity codes in response to Program Announcement (PAs) and Request for Applications (RFAs) in which they participate). Eligibility for the R15 is limited to institutions that have not received more than $6 million per year in NIH support in each of 4 of the last 7 years (see http://grants. nih.gov/grants/funding/area_ineligible.htm). Only NCI and NIEHS offer K22 PAs (no parent announcement); NCI dropped the number of awards from nine to six between FY11 and FY12 (and cut funding for the program by a third as well). While none of these ICs participates in the K01 parent announcement, NCI offers a K01 PA intended to promote diversity (limited to applicants from groups underrepresented in science). Finally, the K99 was not introduced until 2006.

The postdoc would want to consider all of these details in relation to his or her research, eligibility (such as citizenship for the F and K mechanisms and whether his or her institution allows postdocs to submit RPG applications), career status and goals, and institution. The postdoc would then want to search RePORTER (http://projectreporter.nih.gov/reporter.cfm) by keyword for activity codes-IC combinations of most interest. In this case, the

| SEARCH RESEARCH/ DISEASE AREAS | | | | | PRINT | EXPORT | ? | |

Research/Disease Areas (Dollars in millions and rounded)	FY 2008 Actual	FY 2009 Actual	FY 2009 Actual (ARRA)10/	FY 2010 Actual (Non-ARRA)	FY 2010 Actual (ARRA) 10/	FY 2011 Actual	FY 2012 Estimated	FY 2013 Estimated
			(Non-ARRA)					
Acute Respiratory Distress Syndrome	$82	$103	$17	$110	$22	$96	$96	$96
Adolescent Sexual Activity	N/A	N/A	N/A	$80	$7	$69	$69	$69
Agent Orange & Dioxin	$13	$13	$2	$11	$1	$8	$8	$8
Aging	$1,965	$3,015	$554	$2,517	$443	$2,572	$2,562	$2,558
Alcoholism	$452	$441	$75	$454	$65	$452	$454	$452
Allergic Rhinitis (Hay Fever)	$6	$4	$1	$3	$1	$7	$7	$7
ALS	$43	$43	$13	$47	$12	$44	$45	$44
Alzheimer's Disease 12/	$412	$457	$77	$450	$79	$448	$498	$449
American Indians / Alaska Natives	$142	$169	$19	$151	$16	$136	$137	$137
Anorexia	$7	$8	$2	$9	$2	$11	$11	$11
Anthrax	$134	$102	$13	$116	$12	$87	$87	$87
Antimicrobial Resistance	$228	$251	$52	$356	$66	$369	$369	$369
Aphasia	$22	$22	$3	$21	$1	$21	$21	$21
Arctic	$22	$28	$6	$34	$3	$28	$28	$28
Arthritis	$232	$246	$65	$249	$59	$231	$225	$225
Assistive Technology	$215	$249	$43	$250	$48	$250	$250	$250
Asthma	$246	$284	$51	$244	$33	$221	$221	$221
Ataxia Telangiectasia	$13	$13	$2	$12	$1	$13	$13	$13
Atherosclerosis	$460	$495	$112	$544	$104	$475	$475	$474
Attention Deficit Disorder (ADD)	$60	$71	$13	$66	$15	$55	$55	$55
Autism	$118	$132	$64	$160	$58	$169	$169	$170
Autoimmune Disease	$762	$879	$138	$856	$125	$869	$872	$872

FIGURE 6.4   Annual NIH-wide support level for 235 (in 2013) research, condition, and disease categories (http://report.nih.gov/categorical_spending.aspx)

one NIEHS K01 application should certainly be checked, to see what sort of science was funded and to consider the successful Project Summary (abstract) as a model, as well as the 15 NCI K01 awards, paying particular attention to any projects related to DNA repair. With this background information, the postdoc could contact the appropriate career development POs at NIEHS and NCI for advice as to whether to apply for the K01 or an R01 (if the postdoc has sufficient publications to support such an application).

In Table 6.2, note also the growth in the number of applications (while the number of awards has remained roughly the same or declined slightly) over the course of a decade. Your PO(s) will likely have good insight into which mechanisms to favor as well, but these data offer a good starting point, and knowing these in advance of talking with your PO will stand you in good stead. POs like to see you taking some initiative and doing a little background research first, so your conversation can be more meaningful. These are all important decisions to make up front, so be sure to apply your analysis gathering and analysis skills in preparing a long-term application strategy in parallel with your research development.

7

Getting at Mechanism

WHILE UNDERSTANDING THE mechanism of NIH funding is not as critical as understanding the mechanism underlying your disorder of interest, it is very important to developing a successful application strategy. Your research plan must be tailored to the objectives of the funding mechanism and activity code (e.g., R01, F32, K08, etc.). You will know the mechanism before you start preparing your Specific Aims and Research Strategy narratives, but sometimes, you will be repurposing unfunded applications to new activity codes (as explained in Chapter 13), and in these situations especially, you want to ensure that the narrative is modified appropriately.

The NIH distributes funding to extramural researchers through grants and cooperative agreements (contracts are also extramural awards, but they provide specific goods or services to the federal government). A diverse alphabet soup of activity codes (http://grants.nih.gov/grants/funding/ac_search_results.htm) are used, and we will review the major programs and most common funding mechanisms here, including tips for developing non–Research Project Grant (RPG) applications (i.e., career development, fellowship, multiproject programs). Because not all activity codes can be competitively renewed or receive competitive supplements, the award and success rate data are for new (Type 1) applications only. Please note that in several places we include the Web link for the funding announcement associated with a mechanism that was current at the time of this writing but may have since been changed or reissued (see Related Notices box at the outset of the announcement for updates).

Research Grants (R series)

Most of the applications you will submit as principal investigator (PI) will likely be R series proposals, in particular the R01 (with the numeral zero in the middle, not capital letter O).

R01 (3,662 new awards in FY12, 14.9% success rate) (http://grants.nih.gov/grants/funding/r01.htm)

The R01 is the bread-and-butter funding mechanism of the NIH: about half of the extramural awards at the NIH are R01s (25,553 of 51,836 awards issued in FY12), and this is the activity codes Congress tracks in terms of the number of new awards issued. All Institutes and Centers (ICs) except the National Institute on Minority Health and Health Disparities, the National Center for Advancing Translational Sciences, and the Fogarty International Center participate in the parent announcement (at the time of this writing, http://grants.nih.gov/grants/guide/pa-files/PA-13-302.html). Your primary grant-seeking strategy should focus on R01 funding, especially if you are a new or early-stage investigator (ESI).

The R01 is flexible in terms of length (up to 5 years) and budget size (the type of budget used in the application changes at the $250,000 threshold, and applications requesting more than $500,000 in any one year must receive advance permission from the IC for submission). The R01 can be renewed, and it is the one activity code for which new ESI applicants receive a break both in terms of the payline or score threshold for funding decisions and in terms of the award made [budget is cut to a lesser degree, if at all, than for established PIs In addition, applications from new and ESI applicants are reviewed together as a group separate from those of established PIs during study section meetings (Chapter 3), and amended applications (A1s) can be submitted in the same cycle in which they were reviewed, if the PI can revise the proposal within such a short time frame (more on this in Chapter 13). Note that R01 awards can be made to all types of organizations all over the world; there are no citizenship or residency requirements for PIs, although there are special requirements for grants awarded to foreign institutions.

Our grantsmanship advice throughout the book is applicable to R01 applications. You should work with your Program Officer (PO) to refine your aims to fill an important gap in the IC portfolio in a manner that your reviewers will find exciting and compelling (Chapter 3). While the parent announcement will accommodate applications addressing any type of research, you should check your IC and the NIH Guide (http://grants.nih.gov/grants/guide/index.html) to determine whether a Request for Applications (RFA) or Program Announcement (PA) might be appropriate for your work.

With an RFA, you should seek advice from the PO as to whether your proposal would be a good fit—and whether it might fare better in the parent or a broader program announcement. With RFAs, you know the IC has a specific interest in the research objectives listed and that reviewers for these applications will be knowledgeable and excited about the area of research involved. However, if funds are only available for a small number of awards, the competition could be fierce. On the other hand, if you submit an R01 application in response to an RFA but do not receive an award, you can then take advantage of reviewer recommendations and concerns and prepare the same proposal as a new R01 (A0) for the parent or other program announcement. Similarly, you can refine an unfunded A1 from any other Funding Opportunity Announcement (FOA) for submission as an A0 in response to an appropriate RFA.

Due to a Congressional mandate requiring that the average length of an RPG award be 4 years, new and ESI applicants are more likely than established PIs to receive a 5-year award. In recent years, ICs have become more concerned about making long-term obligations due to the volatility and uncertainty in budget negotiations on Capitol Hill, so proposing work that can be accomplished in 3–4 years (more along the National Science Foundation model) rather than trying to fill the traditional 5-year project period may be more attractive to both the IC and the study section. In fact, NHLBI now specifically asks that PIs submit applications requesting 4 years of support (http://www.nhlbi.nih.gov/funding/policies/oper-guid.htm), with a few exceptions (ESI, some clinical trials, AIDS-related research). Of course, the compressed time frame will put more pressure on you in terms of publishing quickly (to demonstrate productivity in time for the next competing renewal) and preparing competing renewal applications more frequently.

Research projects can also be funded as Cooperative Agreements (U01), in which the IC staff has substantial involvement and defined roles. U01 applications are generally solicited through an RFA or Program Announcement Reviewed in an Institute (PAR), and often the PIs of awardee sites serve on a common Steering Committee (or another sort of working or coordinating group) and participate in meetings among program staff and awardees (in person or via teleconference). Sometimes the projects of participating sites are linked (as with consortium research), and sometimes they are independent but focused on a common question or scientific area. Like the R01, the U01 mechanism is quite flexible and can be customized to the needs and priorities of the issuing IC(s). If you respond to a U01 FOA, you will want to work with the PO in planning your proposal and pay close attention to any special application requirements and review criteria.

Please note that you yourself cannot directly apply for some R series awards (hence the tempting 100% success rate), such as the R37 (MERIT or Method to Extend Research in Time) and R56 (High Priority, Short-Term Project) activity code (more on this at the end of the chapter); POs initiate requests for both of these based on a competitively reviewed R01 application.

R21 (1,932 awards, 14.1% success rate) (http://grants.nih.gov/grants/funding/r21.htm)

The next most common R series mechanism is the R21, the NIH Exploratory/Developmental Research Grant Award, is viewed by many to be a "starter" grant. However, due largely to a tremendous increase in the number of applications over the past decade, the success rate for R21s is, in fact, lower than for the R01 (particularly if the much better renewal success rate for Type 2 R01s, 34.6%, is calculated in). Further, only 17 ICs participate in the parent announcement (at time of this writing, http://grants.nih.gov/grants/guide/pa-files/PA-13-303.html). Some of the nonparticipating ICs publish their own PAs for this activity code, but some pretty much eschew the R21 mechanism altogether (e.g., NIGMS, which made 67 awards in FY12, compared with 676 at NIAID or 314 at NHBLI). Many ICs issue PAs using the R21 for research of a specific nature (e.g., pilot studies, clinical trials, secondary data analysis, etc.).

There is no R21 payline break for new or ESI applicants, the award size is limited (generally $275K in direct costs over 2 years), and it cannot be renewed, which is why the NIH generally recommends that junior investigators not use the R21 mechanism as their entrée to independent research support.

The review of R21 applications can be unsatisfying. Study sections, except those devoted to reviewing R21 applications, often struggle with the lack of preliminary data or the high-risk nature (and hopefully high reward) of research proposed. PIs of unsuccessful R21 applications can use reviewer requests for preliminary data that would demonstrate feasibility to prepare an R03 application to collect (and publish) these requested preliminary data and in turn use these data to develop a competitive R01 application. This would be, of course, a very delayed time frame, from the submission of the R21 through the submission, funding, and completion of the R03 project to the submission (and possibly resubmission) and funding of the R01.

R03 (572 awards, 19.9% success rate)
(http://grants.nih.gov/grants/funding/r03.htm)

The Small Research Grant (R03) is exactly that: $50,000 in direct costs per year for 2 years (nonrenewable). The work proposed is time limited and focused, with a clear purpose, such as to collect some pilot data, conduct secondary analyses, or develop an animal model, assay, or other research resource. Less than half of the ICs participate in the parent announcement (http://grants.nih.gov/grants/guide/pa-files/PA-13-304.html); a few offer R03 PAs limited to certain K awardees (since career development awards include very little research funding) or new investigators. For these applications, the key is to propose a manageable, discrete project that will support development of a future R01 or other RPG application.

R13 (378 awards, 60.6% success rate)
(http://grants.nih.gov/grants/funding/r13/index.htm)

For conference awards, you will need to talk with your PO or the IC R13 contact (http://grants.nih.gov/grants/guide/contacts/parent_R13_U13.html) directly. Specifically, you need a letter from the IC R13 PO agreeing to accept your application (you upload this as your cover letter in the electronic application), and input from the PO is especially important since the IC makes these awards with considerable programmatic discretion. These applications are reviewed by an IC rather than CSR study section process, and, while not guaranteed for funding, R13s have a success rate well above 50% at most ICs. Only specific conference costs can be supported with NIH funding, and you should not expect significant funding; check to see your IC cost limits and ask the PO for the typical award size (usually $20K or less).

R15 (177 awards, 13.3% success rate)
(http://grants.nih.gov/grants/funding/area.htm)

Your eligibility to apply for an Academic Research Enhancement Award (AREA) depends on your institution (http://grants.nih.gov/

grants/funding/area_ineligible.htm) or at least your school within a university (e.g., the School of Medicine may not be eligible, but the School of Nursing or Pharmacy might be). The academic component where you have your appointment cannot have received more than $6 million in funding from the NIH for 4 or more of the past 7 years. The award provides $300,000 in direct costs over 3 years and can be renewed. If you are eligible to apply for an R15, you should think of this mechanism as supporting modest R01-type projects with long-term goals that can be achieved in manageable segments. The role of the award in exposing students to research is also important.

R33 (4 awards, 11.4% success rate)

The R33 is the Phase II award for a successful R21 project but is rarely used. Often these applications are solicited through R21/R33 FOAs (NIAID has a sample application and summary statement at http://www.niaid.nih.gov/researchfunding/grant/pages/appsamples.aspx), but ICs sometimes solicit R33 applications on their own (e.g., the NCI Innovative Molecular Analysis Technologies Program, http://imat.cancer.gov). This is an applied, milestone-driven proposal that will include a Gantt chart or other benchmarked timeline laying out the R21 and R33 projects. The milestones (go/no go) must be quantifiable, and you must give sufficient thought to them and the entire timeline; this is often a weakness flagged by reviewers.

R34 (106 awards, 22.9% success rate)
(http://grants.nih.gov/grants/funding/r34.htm)

Although no parent FOA exists for the Clinical Trial Planning Grant Program, many ICs issue their own IC-specific R34 or U34 FOA for multi-site trials. Before applying for an R34, you will want to talk with the appropriate PO about your planned Phase III trial. At some ICs, awards are intended to support the development of data collection tools, operations manual, recruitment strategies, and the final protocol. If it is a multisite trial, this time and funding will allow you to create the infrastructure for communications and data sharing and coordinate protocol submission to the various Institutional Review Boards. At other ICs, this activity code is used to support pilot studies to collect data for use in planning a larger trial.

Small Business Research Project Grant Mechanisms

While small businesses (and other for-profit organizations) can submit applications to most NIH grant mechanisms (check the eligibility information section of the FOA), they can also take advantage of Congressionally mandated programs designed to support the commercialization of discoveries resulting from Federal funding: Small Business Innovation Research (SBIR) and Small Business Technology Transfer (STTR). Keep in mind that the term "small" is relative: applicant businesses can have up to 500 employees.

In FY12, the NIH set aside 0.35% of its budget for STTR (R41/R42) awards and 2.6% of its budget for SBIR (R43/R44) awards. The most recent Congressional reauthorization (http://grants.nih.gov/grants/funding/sbir/reauthorization.htm) of the SBIR program requires that these set-asides be increased to 0.4% in FY14 and 0.45% in FY15 for STTR and to 3.2% by FY17 (via incremental increases of 0.1% per fiscal year) for SBIR.

You will want to bookmark the NIH SBIR Web site (http://grants.nih.gov/grants/funding/sbir.htm) if you will be involved with such applications, and you will want to work closely with the SBIR/STTR PO for your IC in planning and developing your proposal.

STTR: R41 (104 awards, 19.2% success rate)/R42 (39 awards, 37.8% success rate)

With the STTR, you can apply as an employee of either the nonprofit (academic) research institution or the small business. At least 40% of the work (as measured by the direct costs) must be performed by the small business, at least 30% by the nonprofit research institution, and the remaining 30% can be divided among these partners or include a third-party collaborator.

SBIR: R43 (674 awards, 15.8% success rate)/R44 (279 awards, 30.8% success rate) (http://grants.nih.gov/grants/guide/pa-files/PA-13-088.html)

With the SBIR, the contact PI must be primarily employed by the small business, though other PIs as part of a multiple PI application do not. For Phase I awards, the small business must account for at least 67% of the effort, whereas for Phase II awards, this can drop to 50%.

Research Programs (P series)

While the majority of NIH funding supports individual research projects, often the critical mass of independent investigators focused on a common theme exists to support the submission of a Program Project (P01) or Center (P20, P30, P50, P60) grant application. Because the budgets for these awards exceed $500K in direct costs per year, you must obtain permission to submit an application at least 6 weeks prior to the receipt date. In fact, however, ICs would like to see short preproposals (program summary, individual project aims, shared core resources, investigators, etc.) months in advance so that you do not invest significant time and resources preparing an application that your IC is not interested in funding. There is no parent award for any of these activity codes, and the applications are referred to IC review groups (Chapter 2), not to CSR.

For program project applications, the essential ingredient is a unifying theme used to integrate the projects, such that they would not be as effective pursued individually, outside the program. They must feed into and draw on each other. Often aims and data are shared to an extent. ICs vary on whether they want their P01s to be focused on basic science or include a clinical/translational component, but this will become clear in your discussions with the PO and your reading of the IC-specific guidelines. The PIs on each project should be established investigators, though more junior researchers can be involved. ICs and reviewers do not look upon this as a starter mechanism for securing funding for PIs who may not be competitive on their own.

For core center applications, the essential ingredient is a large portfolio of R01 and other awards from the target IC that will be served by the shared resources and services made available through the center. Membership in the center and access to its resources must demonstrate commitment to the currently funded investigators and to expanding the pool of funded investigators, particularly by encouraging new (and nontraditional) researchers to enter this field of research.

For specialized centers of research, the projects should be independent, conducted in parallel, but address a common theme. Projects are can be dually led by a clinical and basic science PI to ensure a translational focus, and in this case, one of the PIs can be more junior, so long as he or she has the requisite scientific expertise and evidence of launching a research career. The cores must directly support all or most of the projects in ways not possible through an institutional core facility. The specialized center mechanisms also support pilot project and career development components intended to launch the next generation of research and researchers in this field.

Career Development (http://grants.nih.gov/training/careerdevelopmentawards.htm)

As with the research project mechanisms, some ICs, either in addition to or instead of participating in the parent announcement, customize one or more career development (K) FOAs, particularly to emphasize diversity in the biomedical research workforce. The key to remember for any K application is that it is not a substitute research project award: you must present a plan for receiving new or specialized training integrated with your proposed project that will allow you to become an independent investigator. Linking your training and mentorship with your research aims in the Candidate section shows that you have thought through how to use the project as a vehicle for any additional training needed and a platform for establishing your independence as a researcher. The K research project should be designed to obtain critical experience and preliminary data for a competitive R01 application.

In addition to seeing through an R01 disguised as a career development application, reviewers will take note if your mentor is a well-funded, well-known scientist but not the right person to oversee your career development. You could have such an individual as part of a mentor team, but your primary mentor, in addition to having a track record of sustained funding and training productive researchers, must be the right person based on your scientific focus. He or she must clearly have the time and genuine commitment to serve as your mentor as well. You should choose wisely, as your need for a mentor does not end when the award does.

You can exploit both the Candidate statement and the Personal Statement on your Biosketch to drive home your preparation for and commitment to a career in biomedical research. You should not hesitate to use the first-person, active voice: it is all about you and what you are doing and what you plan to do. Your background should not just rehash your history but explain your choices, highlight key opportunities you have pursued, and annotate major publications. You want to convey that you have developed your own research question, designed the study to answer it, analyzed the data critically, and interpreted the data both for dissemination and for planning the next phase of research. To demonstrate right off the bat that you know where you are going (and lay the foundation for the recap of how you got to this point), you should start the Candidate section with a statement about your long-term research career goals, including their translational application down the road. Because this is an award to help you complete your preparation for an independent research career, acknowledge any gaps and how your educational and research plans will address them and make you competitive for an R01. If you have no gaps to fill, reviewers will conclude you do not need K funding but should instead move directly to an R01 application (and sometimes, you should).

Reviewers will also look at your publication history to see whether you are prepared to become an independent researcher. You should have some first-author papers from your pre- and postdoctoral training, though clinical scientists may not have had many opportunities to do so. What does not look good are a series of poster presentations that are never completed as manuscripts. Review papers are often discounted as not contributing to a successful K application, but these are no longer the "gimme's" they used to be, especially in good journals, and your preparation of a review in your area of focus demonstrates your commitment to learning the field and a thorough grounding in the background of the scientific problems you seek to address. A reviewer may well take a look-see to gauge your understanding of the field. While original reports give strong indication as to your potential success as a researcher (since others with more data and information available to them will have peer reviewed your science), if you have several first- or last-author original reports, reviewers may wonder whether you need mentored training via K support or are sufficiently prepared to seek independent RPG funding.

Your mentor's statement and letters of collaboration and institutional commitment (from your chair or dean) will be critical, especially if you do not have an academic appointment. These must be personalized and focused on you as a candidate and your proposal, not vague flowery form letters. You should work with your primary mentor on his or her letter and draft letters for other members of your mentoring team and any additional advisors or consultants. The letters must address how the training plan and project will overcome any gaps in your preparation and ensure that you will be competitive for R01 funding and contribute significantly to the field. The primary mentor must show reviewers that he or she is qualified based on a successful track record of funding, publication, and trainees who have moved on to productive independent careers. The letter must convince reviewers that your mentor will be engaged with you and will evaluate your progress (and intervene if you are missing your milestones). The mentor must make a good case for agreeing to serve as your mentor based on his or her assessment of your creativity, commitment, productivity, and potential.

Be sure all the letters agree with the Candidate plan presented in terms of the number and timing of meetings and milestones set. Be sure also to check both the FOA and the SF424 instructions for details on the length, content, and submission process for each required letter.

The project itself, again, should not be a mini-R01. This should be thoughtfully planned to integrate new techniques and collaborations while obtaining preliminary data for a future R01 application (to be submitted during the later years of K support). The idea should be compelling and exciting to reviewers and lead into a long-term program of research, as covered in your goals and objectives. The work itself should encompass an appropriate scope for training and pilot study purposes. For K applications, a "less is more" approach is best. You will demonstrate to reviewers that you understand what is needed and feasible given the time and funding constraints of a K but that will meaningfully contribute to the further development of the research through an R01 application.

Some K activity codes are designed for applicants with clinical degrees (K08, K23, K24), some for basic scientists (K01, K02), some for junior investigators (K01, K08, K23, K25), some for established investigators (K02, K05, K18, K24). The K Kiosk (http://grants.nih.gov/training/careerdevelopmentawards.htm) offers the most current list and descriptions of FOAs in use (some ICs use the same activity code for different purposes). Participation in and success rates for individual FOAs vary widely by IC (http://report.nih.gov/DisplayRePORT.aspx?rid=551), as we illustrated in Chapter 6 in the example of a postdoc trying to decide on a grant strategy, so be sure to do your homework and talk with appropriate K mechanism POs.

Speaking of postdocs, two Career Transition awards limit their eligibility to postdoc applicants: K22 and K99/R00. Only a few ICs offer the K22, and some only for intramural training (at the NIH); some expand eligibility to newly independent faculty as well. You will need the promise of an academic appointment during the award period (for those targeting the postdoc-faculty transition), and you will need to submit an R01 application before the end of the second year (3 years of support).

The K99/R00 (often whimsically called a "kangaroo" after the activity code) was established specifically to decrease the time necessary for talented scientists to become independent investigators. This has met with mixed success, and many ICs are limiting its use. You apply for the K99 mentored career development component as a postdoc (and you can apply without citizenship or permanent residency), so long as you are within 4 years of your terminal degree. The R00 independent research component is activated when you receive a faculty appointment (preferably at an institution other than the one at which you completed the K99 mentored training).

You should note that some applicants have job offers by the time they receive notice of the K99 (whereas ICs want to see a full year of mentored training), and the non-renewable R00 offers $249K in *total* costs, which means institutional indirect costs will eat up a sizeable percentage of the award.

Finally, the K12 is an institutional clinical research career development mechanism for which an established PI submits the application to the NIH; then junior faculty submit applications to the awardee institution competing for the K12 slots (generally from internal candidates but also from external candidates who secure letters of commitment offering a position contingent on receiving a K12 slot). Institutions with a Clinical and Translational Science Award (CSTA, http://www.ncats.nih.gov/research/cts/ctsa/ctsa.html) maintain a KL2 program to support clinical and translational research career development. Both programs offer intensive training and specialized resources (e.g., biostatistical support, grant-writing assistance, reduced core research facility fees, etc.) to participating scholars. Securing a slot on either a K12 or a KL2 program is less competitive than a stand-alone K award, but the support is often limited to 2–3 years—enough time to support the junior faculty member in submitting (and hopefully securing) an appropriate K or R01 application, thus opening the slot for another promising young investigator.

Research Training (http://grants.nih.gov/training/nrsa.htm)

Funding for fellowships and training grants is provided through the National Research Service Award (NRSA) program, which, most of like the career development mechanisms, is only available to citizens, noncitizen nationals, and permanent residents (Green Card must be issued by the time of the award). These are often referred to as Ruth L. Kirschstein National Research Service Awards after a long-time leader at the NIH; see http://www.nih.gov/about/kirschstein/index.htm for a free biography of this remarkable scientist and administrator.

Unlike the K mechanism, postdoctoral trainees supported by F or T mechanisms are required to pay back 1 year of support (http://grants.nih.gov/training/payback.htm). You will not be obligated to pay back more than a year, as each subsequent year of training qualifies as payback for the prior year of support. You can satisfy your payback requirements through continued research or teaching activities but not by patient care. Predoctoral trainees can receive up to 5 years (MD-PhD students can receive up to 6 years of support), and postdoctoral trainees can receive up to 3 years of NRSA support through a combination of F and T mechanisms; altogether, you could receive up to 8 or 9 years of NRSA funding through your pre- and postdoctoral training periods.

The caveats noted earlier for career development applications also apply to fellowships (e.g., proposal should not be an RPG substitute, especially for F32 applications, and the letters and training plans are critical). One F mechanism–specific tip: the electronic application package is one size fits all, which can be tricky. You must be careful that every document relevant to your background and proposal has been uploaded, whether or not it is flagged in the electronic application as required. As always, read the instructions carefully and ask questions as needed.

You might also note that individual fellowships go to CSR study sections but then receive their second level of review within the IC, not by Council (if you look at the parent announcements, the date for Advisory Council Review reads, "Not applicable for Fellowships"). Thus, input from your PO is particularly valuable, both to help ensure your application is sent to the best study section and is framed in a manner that will be attractive to your IC.

If you are involved in an application for an institutional training grant or T32 (these are submitted by an established PI, not by the trainee), the data tables will make or break the application, so be sure to set aside a couple of months to complete them in advance. The faculty and their funding sources are critical, as is the training program as a cohesive whole. The success of past trainees in publishing with their mentors and launching their own independent academic research careers will be a key benchmark for both new and renewing applications. Faculty must have their own independent funding (preferably from the IC to which the T32 application is directed), such that it is clear the T32 is not being used simply to provide additional hands in underfunded research programs.

A Word about Supplements

Administrative supplement applications (http://grants.nih.gov/grants/guide/admin_supp/index.htm) go to your PO and are reviewed and discussed internally. Competitive supplements are full Type 3 applications that are sent to the same study section that reviewed your parent award for which the supplement is sought. Administrative supplements to promote diversity offer you the opportunity to secure funding to support a high school, undergraduate, or graduate student or a postdoc from an underrepresented minority or with a disadvantaged background. You should discuss this with your PO in advance; you will learn through these discussions whether you are likely to be funded (and hence whether to even apply). Competitive revisions (Type 3 applications) had a 24.5% success rate for R01s in FY12. These must propose new aims based on (inspired by) the parent study and cannot simply request additional funds to achieve the originally approved aims.

A Word about Bridge Funding (R56 Awards)

The R56 is not something you apply for; your PO recommends applications for consideration by the IC extramural staff. The R56 is usually for 1 year, sometimes for 2 years, and is not renewable. If your application is of high programmatic priority and just fell outside the funding range, you might suggest to your PO that your project could be pared down to 1 year, focusing on those aims or experiments for which the reviewers showed the greatest enthusiasm and that would have the most impact. The goal would be to obtain data that would then make a new application competitive for full R01 funding. Not many R56 awards are issued (281 total in FY12), so even if your application and score are appropriate, the odds of success are still low, but not zero.

8

Telling Your Story Well

AS WE EXPLAINED in Chapter 3, you need to grab your reviewers' attention on the very first page and tell a compelling story that they want to keep reading. While your science is exciting to you, the key is to convey it in a manner that excites the reviewers and assures them that you are the best investigator to pursue this avenue of research.

Here, we go through the narrative components of the NIH grant application in the order in which we would suggest they be drafted (Chapter 9 briefly reviews the visual and written presentation), starting with the Specific Aims, which may be the only page read by every reviewer on the study section. From there, we move on to the Research Strategy in the order of their contribution to the Overall Impact/Priority Score as demonstrated by analyses by the National Institute of General Medical Sciences (NIGMS) and the Office of Extramural Research (OER).

Please keep in mind throughout that if you have done due diligence in selecting the most appropriate study section (Chapter 3), you can tailor your level of detail and style to the reviewers listed as regular members of the panel, recognizing that you may have an ad hoc reviewer assigned as well. Sending your application to a highly focused Scientific Review Group (SRG) may allow you to jump straight into fundamental questions, with less big-picture overview, but you will need to feel confident that most or all panel members will have this level of a priori understanding.

Also, a quick word on a section no longer formally part of the NIH Research Strategy narrative: *preliminary data*. Whereas the Progress Report for a competing renewal application (Type 2) is included at the outset of the Approach section, preliminary data can be integrated wherever they best strengthen your story. Often they work in the Approach section by demonstrating the feasibility of the proposed method and your ability to obtain good data in support of your hypothesis (then, too, you do not need to repeat unpublished methodological details). However, these data may be more powerful in establishing the significance of the work or the innovation of your approach. While we advise you not to create unnecessary work for reviewers, you can be judicious in succinctly summarizing (and citing) your published findings without repeating figures or extensive detail in the proposal itself.

Finally, a general reminder (from Chapter 3), throughout the entire application, your goal is to make the job of the reviewer as easy as possible (keep in mind the mental image of your reviewer reading the proposal at 2 a.m. with a sick child crying and a pile of his or her own manuscripts and grant applications needing attention). Your goal in how you develop your narrative is to make it efficient—and a pleasure—for the reviewer to read the proposal, present your application to the study section for discussion, and write the bullet points (strengths) in the summary statement. In fact, you should in essence be writing the summary statement bullet points for them.

First, Check the Data

Just as data on funding trends are important in planning your overall application strategy, data on what influences scoring trends are important in developing your individual applications. Analyses of FY10 data, first by NIGMS (https://loop.nigms.nih.gov/index.php/2010/08/09/scoring-analysis-1-year-comparison/) and then by OER for all of the Institutes and Centers (ICs) (https://loop.nigms.nih.gov/index.php/2010/09/30/nih-wide-correlations-between-overall-impact-scores-and-criterion-scores/ and http://nexus.od.nih.gov/all/2011/03/08/overall-impact-and-criterion-scores/, respectively), demonstrate that Approach (based on its individual criterion score), followed by Significance, correlates best with your priority score. This trend holds true across all ICs as shown in Table 8.1 in the correlation coefficients between the overall impact score and the five criterion scores for 32,608 Research Project Grant applications from FY10; while the data have not been presented by SRG, the same would be expected (i.e., emphasis on Approach). This makes sense, of course, since even if the question being addressed is significant, if your proposed method of addressing the question is not robust, the impact will be modest at best.

Table 8.1 Correlation coefficients between the overall impact score and the five criterion scores for 32,608 NIH applications from the FY 10 October, January, and May Council rounds (https://loop.nigms.nih.gov/index.php/2010/09/30/nih-wide-correlations-between-overall-impact-scores-and-criterion-scores/) (please refer to the Abbreviations listing at the outset of the book to identify individual ICs in the first column)

Institute or Center	Approach	Significance	Innovation	Investigator	Environment	No. of Applications with Impact Scores
FIC	0.78	0.59	0.51	0.45	0.54	125
NCCAM	0.78	0.63	0.60	0.60	0.54	285
NCI	0.80	0.67	0.59	0.53	0.45	5,396
NCMHD	0.82	0.69	0.75	0.71	0.57	57
NEI	0.83	0.69	0.62	0.59	0.49	777
NHGRI	0.79	0.69	0.61	0.58	0.52	224
NHLBI	0.82	0.67	0.64	0.56	0.48	3,157
NIA	0.84	0.73	0.65	0.58	0.55	1,521
NIAAA	0.84	0.71	0.63	0.51	0.41	427
NIAID	0.82	0.67	0.62	0.55	0.47	3,809
NIAMS	0.84	0.65	0.65	0.57	0.49	1,051
NIBIB	0.77	0.68	0.63	0.54	0.49	894
NICHD	0.83	0.70	0.63	0.54	0.49	2,074

(continued)

Table 8.1 (Continued)

Institute or Center	Approach	Significance	Innovation	Investigator	Environment	No. of Applications with Impact Scores
NIDA	0.83	0.69	0.60	0.54	0.47	1,230
NIDCD	0.82	0.69	0.58	0.51	0.40	443
NIDCR	0.86	0.70	0.68	0.62	0.54	538
NIDDK	0.83	0.69	0.63	0.60	0.50	2,271
NIEHS	0.83	0.68	0.64	0.56	0.49	490
NIGMS	0.83	0.72	0.63	0.62	0.53	2,856
NIMH	0.80	0.68	0.58	0.50	0.44	1,896
NINDS	0.81	0.67	0.60	0.55	0.49	2,262
NINR	0.83	0.70	0.66	0.59	0.53	260
NCRR	0.81	0.69	0.65	0.59	0.56	426
NLM	0.88	0.74	0.82	0.71	0.67	139
NIH	**0.82**	**0.69**	**0.62**	**0.56**	**0.49**	**32,608**

The data are cut many different ways at the NIGMS and OER Web sites noted earlier, but these correlation coefficients provide the most relevant guidance in telling your story.

Specific Aims

You should write the Specific Aims first—and revise this page multiple times over the course of developing the rest of the narrative. The Specific Aims page drives the rest of the application, so you must get this right before you can proceed to the Research Strategy. This will be the only page that many (if not most) reviewers on the study section will read, so it must summarize all the key details: why the work is important, what problem will you solve, why are you the one to solve it, how will you do so, and what the impact will be. This is why you will need to keep revisiting your early versions to update them as details are added or modified later in the Research Strategy.

The Specific Aims page will set the tone for your entire application in the minds of your reviewers. You want that response to be "Wow" rather than "Okay…" (and definitely not, "Huh?").

What you seek to achieve is a convincing case that your science, pursued in the manner that you propose, by you and your team specifically, will meaningfully advance the field. Your science must be something your reviewers will want to read about in the literature in the years ahead. Here is officially what reviewers must consider when assigning their overall impact/priority score:

> *Reviewers will provide an overall impact/priority score to reflect their assessment of the likelihood for the project to exert a sustained, powerful influence on the research field(s) involved.*

The science could be very important, but if reviewers have doubts whether the approach you propose or the team you assemble is the best to move the field toward this exciting end, your score will suffer. We will talk in the next section about the Approach, but first you should concentrate on distilling and capturing both the specific message of your science and the meta-message of your proposal as a whole on one page, the Specific Aims page.

Remembering again that reviewers will not devote time to parsing through dense language full of abbreviations and jargon (your reviewers will not all be experts familiar with your terms and concepts), you want the story to flow easily, capturing the key concepts and entire story line while not getting hung up on detail. It can be difficult to consider what information is most important to convey and what can be left for later in the narrative. Starting with a bare bones rendition and fleshing out the story as you have room is a good strategy. You might want to send out the bare bones version to colleagues, your Program Officer (PO), and anyone else who can help you refine the story; the questions they ask will give you a fresh and outside perspective on what details reviewers might find most useful and important.

Repeating a lot of broad well-known facts at the outset can waste precious real estate on the page and could send the signal that this is a routine story. The first sentence should prepare the reviewer for the ultimate point of the research proposed—not necessarily jumping straight into the hypothesis, though this strategy can work in some cases—something that helps the reviewer know right off the bat where you are going. You want to grab their attention by establishing the scope of the problem (morbidity/mortality/cost/broad fundamental impact) and the gap in our knowledge that your work will fill.

Although there is no one "best" formula for how to develop your Specific Aims narrative, roughly speaking, within the first (short) paragraph, you should lay out the significance of the problem being addressed, the product of the research, rather than the process of producing it. Established investigators and principal investigators (PIs) submitting competing renewals can feature their prior contributions to the literature in conveying the significance of the research.

The second paragraph should bring you into the picture by integrating your take on the problem based on the available literature and how your prior work and preliminary data for this proposal move the story forward. By the end, reviewers should agree with you as to the scientific junction reached and the need to take the next step in the direction you suggest.

The third paragraph lays out your hypothesis and your overall approach to addressing it. At this point, you introduce your specific aims.

Now, whether you have used separate paragraphs to communicate all this depends on your style and how much you need to present. You want to be sure it flows logically, which is where outside readers will be most helpful. Some applicants include a diagram on the Specific Aims page. This can be a powerful communication tool if appropriate for the work and designed properly. If it merely repeats what is in the text or cannot be understood at a glance, your space is probably better reserved for a carefully crafted narrative.

The aims themselves are critical. They need to include enough information for study section members who do not read your Research Strategy to understand how you will pursue these aims. They need to make it easy for your primary reviewer to present and advocate for your application.

There is no "correct" number of specific aims, though keep in mind that most ROIS are now typically limited to 4 years, such that proposing four or more aims may stretch the feasibility of your story. You should be sufficiently familiar with your methods to know how long it will take to complete complicated experiments, accrue eligible patients, breed or obtain animals with the right genotype, prepare special reagents, and so on. Your reviewers will be familiar with all this, and they will expect you to demonstrate your qualifications for the research in proposing a body of work that is logically organized and can manageably be completed in the time allotted. If not, they may have doubts about whether you have sufficient experience. That is, the manner in which you frame your project may suggest you have not encountered the difficulties typical for that type of study and therefore may not be able to pull off the work proposed; this also comes out in how you handle the potential pitfalls piece of the Approach.

A general grantsmanship mnemonic is to develop SMART aims: specific, measurable, attainable, relevant, time-based. Reviewers will assess your competence as a scientist based on the aims you propose: whether they can be achieved in the time appropriate for the funding mechanism and will be clearly achieved (fishing expeditions and observational studies lack an obvious goal line or benchmark for successful attainment). The aims should be complementary but not conditional, and they must generate information useful to the field, whether or not they support your underlying hypothesis. Your aims should flow sequentially but should be capable of being pursued in parallel to a certain extent (that is, as noted earlier, they should not be conditional). As much as possible, they should clearly state the product of the work proposed, with just enough detail for the reviewers to concur that your means of achieving this end are appropriate and, indeed, optimal.

No one best practice will work for everyone since your aims must be customized to the science and the funding announcement and according to whether the work is hypothesis-driven or applied. Our recommendation is to discuss your aims while you are still developing them with as many people as possible. It is best to get these right before you start putting work into writing up the Approach. If the aims change down the line, sometimes it is hard to give up a sexy experiment or technique you included for an earlier version of the aims that is no longer appropriate for the revised aims (or you just neglect to go back and make the change due to deadline constraints).

We will take advantage of sample applications made available online by the National Institute of Allergy and Infectious Diseases (NIAID) (http://www.niaid.nih.gov/researchfunding/grant/Pages/appsamples.aspx) to illustrate some of the points we have made here. Common among these is the limited use of abbreviations and acronyms and the conceptualization of the science in accessible language. Even if a reviewer is not an expert in the PI's field, he or she would feel comfortable reading and following the story being presented.

Two of the sample R01 applications received impact/priority scores of 10, both submitted by early-stage investigator (ESI) applicants. One is the first submission (A0), while the other is a second revision (A2) submitted during the final year such applications were accepted (last regular submission date was November 5, 2010).

The A0 application (http://www.niaid.nih.gov/researchfunding/grant/Documents/Wahlbyresplan.pdf), entitled *Image analysis for high-throughput C. elegans infection and metabolism assays*, is from Dr. Carolina Wahlby (Broad Institute). She summarizes the challenge, approach, and impact of each aim, recaps the overall goal and significance, and includes a few lines at the bottom identifying the names, affiliations, and contributions of her major collaborators; this last addition is helpful for those reviewers who will not go beyond the Specific Aims page to know she, an ESI applicant, does have a strong team capable of achieving what is proposed. She does not load up the page with jargon or procedural detail but does clearly communicate exactly what they will do and why it is important. The Resume and Summary of Discussion of her summary statement (http://www.niaid.nih.gov/researchfunding/grant/Documents/WahlbySS.pdf) confirms the many strengths of her proposal, all of which can be gleaned from the Specific Aims page alone.

The A2 application (http://www.niaid.nih.gov/researchfunding/grant/Documents/Ratnerresplan.pdf), entitled, *Gardnerella vaginalis: toxin production and pathogenesis*, is from Dr. Jonathan Ratner (Columbia University). He takes a very simple and streamlined approach of writing one paragraph addressing the significance, overall goals, and individual aims of the research and lists very succinct specific aims and sub-aims, filling the bottom third of the page with a schema summarizing the flow and substance of the experimental design, resources used, and anticipated outcomes. In the summary statement, the reviewers acknowledge his responsiveness to their prior critique (http://www.niaid.nih.gov/researchfunding/grant/Documents/RatnerSS.pdf), but the emphasis is on the strengths of the work proposed and the excitement generated among the panel.

Although neither of these applications do so, you can make your reviewers' job even easier by concluding with a paragraph labeled "Overall Impact" that summarizes the take-home message you will want your primary reviewer to use in presenting your application. Here is your opportunity to specifically and clearly state how your team conducting the research proposed will "exert a sustained, powerful influence" on your field and advance the public health mission of the NIH. Here is where you say what will be possible after your research has been completed that is not possible or known now.

Approach

Are the overall strategy, methodology, and analyses well-reasoned and appropriate to accomplish the specific aims of the project? Are potential problems, alternative strategies, and benchmarks for success presented? If the project is in the early stages of development, will the strategy establish feasibility and will particularly risky aspects be managed?

Once you have your Specific Aims page in good shape, you will want to concentrate on presenting a clean, compelling approach to clearly achieve these aims—and provide useful data even if the outcome is not what you anticipate. In doing so, you want to be sure you have made it easy for reviewers to assess the assigned review criteria (in italics at the beginning of this section).

A modular approach based on your aims will allow reviewers to quickly see you have addressed all the key review criteria in a parallel fashion. For each aim, you could briefly restate the rationale and hypothesis, integrate relevant preliminary data, succinctly summarize the design and individual experiments (as sub-aims, as appropriate), and conclude with your analysis plan, interpretation of the results, and potential problems and alternative approaches.

For studies in which one central study is designed to answer multiple questions (such as a clinical trial), you would probably present a unified Approach for the entire study (for basic research, this might be a general methods section), breaking down the outcomes and questions to be answered in the anticipated results section. You would then conclude the Approach section with a summary of how this work would be continued toward achieving your long-term goals.

The key is to break down the task and present your approach in a manner appropriate to the science, which in itself will help reassure reviewers that you are thinking about the problem clearly and logically. Illustrating your approach, particularly the underlying theoretical or study design model, in a figure could be well worth the space invested.

Given the page limitations, your focus should not be on the procedural minutiae but on the overall study design and goal of each experiment, with key methodological detail (animal model, cell lines, custom reagents and assays, etc.) included by name. Anything that is published can be cited: your application of established (published) methods to the problem at hand is what reviewers will want to understand. Any of your publications that demonstrate the feasibility of these methods in your hands are especially important. Again, complex, integrated experiments (within or across aims) might best be conveyed by appropriate diagrams.

In applications with clinical studies, you will want to be very clear and complete in describing your cohort (demographics, inclusion/exclusion criteria), your recruitment strategy, and your plans for minimizing and handling dropouts. You must have precise primary and secondary outcome measures and appropriate (validated) tools for measuring each. The statistical analysis will be critical, and reviewers will know if a biostatistician has worked with you on developing the proposal (a statistician is generally assigned as a reviewer). The analytic approach must be consistent with the aims and must clearly answer the questions set forth.

In fact, the data analysis section must be strong for any type of research, and you should indicate how you will interpret the data, whether they are or are not what you anticipate, and what additional steps you might need to take to better understand the initial observations or to modify your approach to address your hypothesis, in case the data are not clear. Reviewers take seriously the anticipated results, potential pitfalls, and alternative approaches sections for each aim (and the overall study), so it should not be just an afterthought or a restatement of what you expect to observe.

Going back to the NIAID sample applications, Dr. Ratner's R01 (http://www.niaid.nih.gov/researchfunding/grant/Documents/Ratnerresplan.pdf) lays out for each subaim the Experimental Design; Anticipated Results and Interpretation; and Potential Pitfalls, Alternative Approaches, and Future Directions. The Anticipated Results text does not simply repeat what he hypothesized would happen but also addresses the significance of the findings in the context of the current body of knowledge and how they will advance the field (impact). The Potential Pitfalls section reassures reviewers that even if experiments do not play out as anticipated, the data will be useful, and the overall body of work can proceed as planned regardless. Indeed, the study section specifically applauded Dr. Ratner for his "innovative approaches which are reflected by a logical flow of the experimental plan."

Overall, reviewers are looking to see that you understand how to apply the tools and techniques appropriately to precisely and unambiguously answer the questions posed and that you will be able to analyze and interpret your data and use them to advance your ongoing body of research. When preparing any grant application, consider the proposed work in the context of a 10-year plan. You want to convey to reviewers that you are looking not just to complete a single project (as would have been the case in your graduate student or postdoc days) but to launch or continue an independent research career (including starting a new line of study, for established investigators).

Significance

Does the project address an important problem or a critical barrier to progress in the field? If the aims of the project are achieved, how will scientific knowledge, technical capability, and/or clinical practice be improved? How will successful completion of the aims change the concepts, methods, technologies, treatments, services, or preventative interventions that drive this field?

As shown in Table 8.1, Significance plays the next largest role in driving Overall Impact/Priority Score. To help reviewers distinguish Significance from Overall Impact, OER convened a working group to write up guidance on this task (http://grants.nih.gov/grants/peer/guidelines_general/impact_significance.pdf). Unlike Overall Impact, the evaluation of Significance assumes the aims of the projects will be achieved, with the question being whether their successful completion will advance the field. In other words, assuming everything goes according to plan, is the research important?

Unfortunately, many applicants still write this section as they did the "Background" or "Background and Rationale" section in the old application format. The Significance section should not be a mini-review paper or a tutorial for reviewers. Instead, you want to focus on why your central question or concepts are important to address—the precise gap in our knowledge that must be filled. You might even divide the content of your Significance section under subheadings such as "Importance of the Problem" and "Knowledge to Be Gained" (or "Impact on the Field") based on the review criteria (presented in italics at the beginning of this section).

If you have heeded the advice in Chapter 3 and know your study section roster as you prepare this section, you can take into consideration which perspectives your potential reviewers will bring when scoring the significance of your work. While you need not cite all their papers, you should keep them in mind when framing this portion of the narrative and the project overall.

The length of your Significance section will depend on the complexity and creativity of your proposal and whether you want to incorporate some of your own preliminary data here. Having colleagues review this section will help you gauge whether you are making a compelling case that your project needs to be done.

Your job in the Significance, then, is to build desire for your project. It is not there to showcase how smart or well read you are, though new investigators often feel compelled to "prove" themselves here. It is there to give a compelling answer to the question: why does this project deserve scarce funding dollars?

Innovation

Does the application challenge and seek to shift current research or clinical practice paradigms by utilizing novel theoretical concepts, approaches or methodologies, instrumentation, or interventions? Are the concepts, approaches or methodologies, instrumentation, or interventions novel to one field of research or novel in a broad sense? Is a refinement, improvement, or new application of theoretical concepts, approaches or methodologies, instrumentation, or interventions proposed?

If Significance is intended to convey why your work is important to do, Innovation should convey why your aims and approach are different from and better than current approaches being taken.

This is another tricky review criterion, as the methods need not be innovative for the research to make exciting discoveries. Reviewers who are sold on your science may acknowledge that the methods are not new but are appropriate for the study to succeed and bring innovative findings to the field. You can help with this distinction by labeling your paragraphs "Technical Innovation" and "Conceptual Innovation."

If you are in fact developing a new method or resource as part of the work proposed, you may need more space for Innovation. Generally, though, no more than a few paragraphs are needed, as the science itself should speak to its innovativeness. However, in the vein of making life easy for your reviewers, you could include a summary sentence or bullet point (or more than one as appropriate) clearly stating how your work advances the field in a way not possible without departing from the status quo as you have proposed.

Introduction

If you are submitting a revised application (A1), you will need to prepare a one-page response (a few mechanisms allow longer responses) to the prior review, which is called the Introduction in NIH grant applications. Many PIs consider this their "rebuttal," which can turn into "debate." However, you should remember that the reviewer is always right. Often it is best if you write what you really want to tell reviewers based on your initial visceral reaction and then run that version through a shredder...multiple times, if needed. Furthermore, keep in mind that the reviewers of your revised application may be different from those who reviewed your original submission. Thus, you want to take on the big issues raised by the review and not get into a passionate discussion of a minor point raised by a single reviewer. If you feel one reviewer in particular includes factual errors in his or her critique, you can ask in your cover letter that the Scientific Review Officer (SRO) not reassign this particular reviewer, but this decision is at the discretion of the SRO. Sometimes your harshest critics can become your biggest fans on resubmission.

Once you are in the proper frame of mind, focus on the concerns raised in the Resume and Summary of Discussion, since the entire panel agreed that these needed to be addressed to increase their collective enthusiasm (and lower their collective score); individual reviewers do not always go back to revise comments in their individual critiques that were adequately resolved during the discussion. You are best off quoting any weaknesses verbatim rather than paraphrasing. With a direct quote, there is no risk of misinterpreting, minimizing, or exaggerating a specific point, which could serve merely to irritate and possibly raise new concerns in the mind of an A1 reviewer. In terms of format, a bulleted or indented style helps quickly move the reviewer through your responses and major changes.

With only a page, you do not want to waste space (or reviewer patience) quoting praise from the prior summary statement or restating other obvious details readily obtained from the application package. While you do not want to go on at length, a brief appreciative acknowledgment of the panel's time and expertise in reviewing and leading to the improved revision of your application is polite. Often a sentence to this effect combined with an explanation of how changes to the revised narrative have been marked or highlighted is all you need to start the Introduction. After that, you want to get right to the point, which is how you have strengthened the proposal since your last submission.

In addressing each concern raised, you want to succinctly provide (depending on what is appropriate to your situation) how you have addressed the point upon resubmission and how the concern has been resolved in the revised narrative—or why it has not. Do not ignore any of the concerns listed in the Resume and Summary of Discussion or raised individually by two or more reviewers (especially important if your Ao was not discussed).

If you have new data or a new manuscript accepted or published that helps establish your response to a concern, by all means highlight this here and cite the section in the narrative where details can be found. The same is true if you have added a new collaborator with expertise that the reviewers felt was missing from the original submission. Ditto for an animal model or assay established during the intervening months (with either a publication or preliminary data to show feasibility). If a paper by another group published since you last submitted helps make your case, you can highlight this as well.

Often your PO will be willing to review your Introduction and Specific Aims, and you should take advantage of any willingness to do so, since your PO likely knows the study section "culture" and reviewer preferences. As usual, having anyone not familiar with your project review both the Resume and Summary of Discussion and your response will offer good insight into what you are actually communicating and the tone and manner in which you are doing so. In fact, if possible, you should ask a colleague or two to read your summary statement and list what they interpret as the major concerns and how these would be best addressed before showing them your Introduction. If you start off making the wrong assumptions, your response and revision will be flawed.

Protection of Research Subjects (Human, Animal)

Your Approach section must contain essential details about any research involving humans and/or vertebrate animals, of course, but what you write for these components of the application is also taken into account when the score is assigned (also if you must address any biohazards in the work proposed). The process of preparing these sections may trigger you to go back and flesh out a particular detail in the Approach that might have otherwise slipped your attention, too.

The NIAID has resources to help you decide whether you are conducting research involving human subjects (including stem cells) and how to prepare the required documents if so (http://www.niaid.nih.gov/researchfunding/

sci/human/Pages/default.aspx). The National Heart, Lung, and Blood Institute likewise offers a Clinical Research Guide (http://www.nhlbi.nih.gov/crg/index.php), including specific guidance on preparing the Human Subjects Protection components of the NIH application (http://www.nhlbi.nih.gov/crg/app_section-e.php). The National Institute on Aging Clinical Research Toolbox (http://www.nia.nih.gov/research/dgcg/clinical-research-study-investigators-toolbox/startup) gives templates and advice on preparing the documents needed for a clinical trial. You should also check the guidelines given to reviewers (http://grants.nih.gov/grants/peer/guidelines_general/Human_Subjects_Protection_and_Inclusion.pdf).

The NIAID also provides an excellent resource to help with your Vertebrate Animals component (http://www.niaid.nih.gov/researchfunding/sci/animal/pages/anitutorial.aspx). You can also read the reviewer checklist (http://grants.nih.gov/grants/olaw/VASchecklist.pdf) for your Vertebrate Animals section to be sure you have provided all the required information. The NIH Office of Laboratory Animal Welfare offers guidance on preparing animal study protocols (http://grants.nih.gov/grants/olaw/sampledoc/animal_study_prop.htm), but this level of detail is more appropriate for your protocol submission to the IACUC (Institutional Animal Care and Use Committee) at your institution than for the Vertebrate Animal section of your NIH application. An often overlooked component of proposing animal research is the required sample size calculations to confirm you are using the correct number of animals (enough to obtain significant results but not excessive use).

How you respond to the required questions for each of these sections will also convey to reviewers your comfort with and competence in conducting clinical or in vivo research. You want them to be reassured that you are aware of and ready to handle any issues you could encounter. Remember, the Overall Impact reflects reviewers' confidence in you and your team in terms of your likelihood to achieve your stated aims and in turn have a significant impact on your field.

Project Summary

You will want to write your Project Summary (abstract) last to ensure it reflects your final version, though an initial draft for your PO may help at the outset in developing your aims and approach. The Project Summary is the public face of your research, if it receives an award, and, along with the Specific Aims, is one of the few pieces of your application that you can expect all reviewers on the study section to read.

If you do not include a cover letter (though we absolutely encourage you to routinely prepare one), this is what the Center for Scientific Review (CSR) referral officers will use in deciding which IC to assign as primary or secondary and to which study section your application should be sent for review. Even if you request a specific study section in your cover letter, the SRO will review your abstract and specific aims to determine whether to accept your application or ask the CSR to make a different assignment.

In other words, this is not a throw-away 30 lines of text. This first impression may become the sole basis on which some reviewers judge your credibility, the novelty and significance of your project, the soundness of your approach, and the impact on your long-term research program and the field as a whole.

Other Application Components

Investigator(s). *Are the PD/PIs, collaborators, and other researchers well suited to the project? If Early-Stage Investigators or New Investigators, or in the early stages of independent careers, do they have appropriate experience and training? If established, have they demonstrated an ongoing record of accomplishments that have advanced their field(s)? If the project is collaborative or multi-PD/PI, do the investigators have complementary and integrated expertise; are their leadership approach, governance, and organizational structure appropriate for the project?*

Environment. *Will the scientific environment in which the work will be done contribute to the probability of success? Are the institutional support, equipment, and other physical resources available to the investigators adequate for the project proposed? Will the project benefit from unique features of the scientific environment, subject populations, or collaborative arrangements?*

You do not want to neglect narrative components of the application that often get short shrift, such as the Personal Statement of your Biosketch or the Facilities and Other Resources file, each of which contributes to the individual criterion scores for Investigator(s) and Environment, respectively.

To convey that you and the other investigators are the best team to conduct the proposed research, you will want to be sure your Personal Statements are detailed, integrated, and focused on the currently proposed project (not cut and paste from another application). You do not want to recapitulate achievements listed elsewhere on the Biosketch but instead tell a story about how your experience to date led to this particular proposal, including your interactions with collaborators on the application. This should be written in the first person, and it can include personal (subjective) information relevant to your motivation and expertise that might not be apparent from your positions, awards, and publications.

Similarly, you do not want your collaborators to give short shrift to their letters of support. They not need be lengthy, but they do need to convey more than a passing familiarity with and pro forma enthusiasm for the project. This is another opportunity to highlight the impact of your work and how well you will work together as a team—and for career development awards, how the research and career of the PI will be advanced through your interaction.

Junior faculty applicants will want to highlight institutional commitment (your startup package) in the Facilities and Other Resources section, and your may want to consider a letter of support from their chair confirming for reviewers that the Department is enthusiastic about your work and committed to seeing you succeed.

If appropriate, your Multiple PI Plan (http://grants.nih.gov/grants/multi_pi/overview.htm) will likewise contribute to your Investigator(s) score and must convince reviewers that the science drives the need for more than one PI and that your collaborative plan will ensure the smooth conduct of the project and dissemination of results.

Your Resource Sharing Plans do not affect your impact score but must be adequate, or your application will be flagged with administrative concerns. The NIAID offers examples of Data Sharing and Model Organism Sharing Plans (http://www.niaid.nih.gov/researchfunding/grant/Pages/samples.aspx). You can also find guidance (http://gwas.nih.gov/06researchers1.html) and sample data-sharing plans (http://gwas.nih.gov/pdf/gwas_data_sharing_plan.pdf) for genome-wide association studies (GWAS).

Cover Letter

It is always to your benefit to include the optional cover letter, which is in fact required for certain applications: those with annual direct costs exceeding $500,000, R13/U13 applications, late or corrected applications, and applications for which videos will be submitted after the application is referred for review (http://grants.nih.gov/grants/guide/notice-files/NOT-OD-12-141.

html). The optional cover letter can be used to request referral to one or more ICs and assignment to a specific SRG, and you can list both specific individuals who should not be assigned your application to review (e.g., the names of competitors or individuals with whom you have had long-standing issues) and the type of expertise assigned reviewers should have (but not names).

You will lay these out as bullet points, with one request per line, followed by a short narrative explanation justifying each (the SF424 Application Guide, http://grants.nih.gov/grants/funding/424/index.htm, includes an example). For the IC request(s), you can cite the PO(s) with whom you have communicated about the application in advance (this also gives the SRO a heads-up on whom to contact if he or she has any questions). The rationale for excluding specific individuals must be based on objective evidence, such as grant awards or publications that clearly demonstrate direct competition; you cannot ask to exclude a reviewer because he or she was mean to you at a poster session.

As noted earlier, without a cover letter, the CSR referral office will need to read your abstract and possibly your Specific Aims (and hopefully nothing else) to determine the best IC and SRG for your application. However, you should strategically make these decisions and develop your application accordingly rather than letting its assignment become one based on the brief attention paid by a referral officer not as familiar with your work as you are.

Budget

Although consideration of the budget and project period does not affect the impact score, reviewers do need to evaluate whether the requested amounts are appropriate for the research proposed. With modular budgets (http://grants.nih.gov/grants/funding/modular/modular.htm), which are used for most R01, R03, R15, R21, and R34 applications with annual direct costs of $250,000 or less (plus some RFAs and PARs), there is less for reviewers to consider, though they might comment on the number of modules ($25K each) requested or the justification of personnel on the project. Applications that involve a foreign institution (either as the applicant or a subaward), R01 applications with direct costs above $250K, and mechanisms not noted earlier must use a nonmodular (detailed) budget.

Both sets of budget forms are included as "Optional" forms in the electronic SF424 application package you will download from the funding opportunity announcement (FOA). You must move the correct set of forms over to complete (the budget itself is not optional). You will need budget-related details specific to your institution, in particular the Facilities and Administrative (F&A) or "indirect" cost rate and the basis on which it is calculated. Indirect costs are specific to each applicant institution and are based on the cost of space and doing research there. Institutions that have built new buildings will be able to negotiate higher indirect cost rates (this is nothing you do).

Your department, school, or institution should have a qualified fiscal administrator who can help develop the budget according to institutional policy; unfortunately, we cannot provide specific guidance on this except to note that you want to propose the appropriate costs for the work to be done. That is, you should not try to include a budget that is clearly too low for the project, as reviewers will be familiar with the research approach and may take your inability to estimate the costs correctly as a reflection of your lack of experience with the work to be done. On the other hand, you will also not get away with padding your budget in anticipation of the budget cut that will inevitably be imposed at the time of award (see Chapter 14). The study section will recommend cuts if your request is not in line with the typical costs and effort involved.

Grant Application Writing Resources

- NIAID Grant Tutorials: http://www.niaid.nih.gov/researchfunding/ grant/pages/aag.aspx
- NIAID Samples and Examples: http://www.niaid.nih.gov/ researchfunding/grant/pages/samples.aspx
- NIMH Grant Writing and Approval Process: http://www.nimh.nih. gov/research-funding/grants/writing-approval-process/index.shtml
- NINDS How to Write a Research Project Grant Application: http:// www.ninds.nih.gov/funding/write_grant_doc.htm

9

Presenting Your Message Well

FORMATTING THE NARRATIVE portions of your application may seem like a trivial detail, but you might consider the manner in which your text is organized, formatted (beyond adhering to font and formatting restrictions in the application instructions), and presented could affect your review. While no single approach to style or format is best, and two reviewers of the same application could have complete opposite preferences, we suggest some overarching considerations to keep in mind when laying out the text, perhaps the most important of which is that reviewers would generally prefer more white space over more words.

Organizing Your Ideas

In the vein of making life as easy as possible for the reviewer, you should use an organizational scheme that ties the major proposal sections together within and across the major application headings (Specific Aims, Significance, Innovation, Approach). You can and should, when possible and as appropriate, incorporate review criteria in your subheadings, so reviewers can quickly find the points in your narrative that satisfy these criteria. For example:

- Under Significance, "Importance of Problem Addressed," "Importance of Knowledge to Be Gained," and "Impact on the Field"
- Under Innovation, "Technical Innovation," "Conceptual Innovation," and "Translational Innovation"

With the shorter application length, you generally do not need to impose a complex alpha-numeric numbering system on your narrative paragraphs. Bold paragraph headings (with no numbering) and judicious use of white space should be sufficient for most applications.

The Approach should be broken down by Specific Aim and by subaim, as appropriate (see Chapter 8). As just noted, you probably will not need additional paragraph numbering, as your narrative will be streamlined enough to allow any necessary cross-referencing by Specific Aim. However, some applications may still benefit from limited numbering to add clarity in cross-referencing, so simply apply good judgment and seek feedback from colleagues as to whether they can follow the flow of your message.

You will want to keep paragraphs short to move the reader quickly through the text and, as noted at the outset, enforce the inclusion of white space so the application can "breathe." No reviewer wants to encounter a solid block of text page after page, and if you cannot comfortably communicate your concept and approach within the space allotted, perhaps you either need to think through and better refine your ideas or tackle less in your proposal.

You can also help the reader move through your ideas by using topic sentences to preview each concept or approach taken (more later on the science of communicating) and by incorporating well-designed graphics that convey important but complex ideas without repeating material written in the text. To help the reviewer's eye easily and quickly go between figures and tables and the point in the text where they are discussed, you should set the in-line reference to these in bold typeface [e.g., **Figure 3 (B)** or **Table 2**].

Reader-Friendly Formatting

Although every aspect of your science may be exciting and high impact and ALL CAPS worthy to you, you want to be kind to your reader, who prefers that his or her attention be drawn stylistically only to the two to three most critical points on the page. During the discussion of your application, limited use of visually imposed emphasis (i.e., bold, italicized, or underlined text) will help reviewers who have not read your application quickly find such key points. If everything is highlighted, the impact is lost, as is readability.

Remember that underlining was used during the typewriter era before type could be easily italicized; some reviewers may feel that underlining should have gone out with the typewriter. Used judiciously and sparingly (a few words at a time), underlined text helps provide emphasis. Used too much or for too long a stretch, it makes the text difficult to read and deadens the sensitivity of reviewer to the import of the message.

Bold typeface is generally the most appropriate way to highlight section or paragraph headings, while italics can be added to visually indicate a change in hierarchy, such as from major to minor subheadings. Bold typeface in the narrative itself is best reserved to help the reader make connections with items elsewhere in the proposal, such as when calling out figures or tables (see earlier) or cross-referencing a Specific Aim.

The key point is here, again, is that any method you use to emphasize text will be a bit harder on the eye to read, so you do not want to burden the reviewers or desensitize them to what is truly important and worthy of notice by overusing bold, italic, or underlined type. Rather, white space can both serve as a method of emphasis and draw the reviewers' attention to essential points being made, since they will not be buried in a wall of text.

Something else to consider in terms of being kind to your reader and enhancing readability: although full justification (flush right and left margins) looks clean and impressive when looking down at the page, the spacing artificially inserted to make the flush margins possible can carry a penalty in readability to the human eye. Your eye also uses the ragged right margin to help keep your place on the page. You cannot predict your reviewers' preferences in this regard, but the science of reading suggests that text with a ragged right margin will be more easily followed by a tired reader.

For resubmission (A1) applications, you need to highlight revised text unless you note in the Introduction that the entire proposal has been substantially revised, such that changes are not marked, and this same formatting advice applies. You will not want to use bold, italicized, underlined, shaded, or colored typeface. Reader-friendly options include vertical lines in the margin or a different font; for example, if you use a sans-serif font such as Arial for your main text, switch to a serif font such as Palatino Linotype or Georgia for your revised text. You will point out in your Introduction how the changes can be recognized, so you must remember to be consistent (and complete) in modifying the presentation of revised or new material.

Now, reviewer preference for the font you select (from among those allowed for NIH applications) or your endnote citation style (numeric versus author-year) varies widely, and you will always make one camp happy at the expense of another. You should make these formatting decisions based on what works well for you (and does not raise criticism or concern among your pre-submission reviewers) and not be too concerned with debates focused on such fine details. You do not want to make the application difficult to follow through cumbersome formatting, but as long as your message is clear and easily followed, your science determines the merit rather than the typeface.

Science of Communicating

In addition to the science you are communicating to the reviewer, there is a science of how you communicate this information. Highly complex science writing need not be impenetrable. Your goal is to place the information where the brain expects to find it and to guide your readers to interpret what you write as you intend them to. A few key points to keep in mind:

- Minimize the separation between subject and verb—do not burden the reviewer to keep track of these by separating them by multiple or lengthy descriptive phrases.
- Articulate the direction action in the verb if appropriate (e.g., "X inhibits the expression of Y" rather than "Y expression is X dependent," which would leave the reviewer wondering exactly how X affects the expression of Y).
- The subject whose story is being told should be at the beginning of the sentence in the topic position (e.g., whether the sentence should read "Bees disperse pollen" or "Pollen is dispersed by bees" depends on whether the rest of the paragraph is about bees or pollen, respectively).
- New, important (exciting!) information should be at the end of the sentence in the stress position; the reader perceives this information as worthy of emphasis, whereas information buried in the middle is not as readily absorbed (reader may need to go back to review it upon completing the sentence).
- The topic position (beginning) of a sentence should include information from the prior sentence that links backward and provides context in moving forward to prevent the reader from getting lost as a complex idea is developed.

Consider too that research is an active endeavor. The experiments are not doing themselves. Although formal science communication has traditionally emphasized third-person passive prose, such a style, in addition to being wordy, does not generate excitement or suggest impact. You should try to use active rather than passive voice, in which case the first person ("I" or "we") is appropriate.

You can also maintain the energy and excitement through short, concise sentences, which are much easier for a reviewer to digest (especially after midnight) than long, complex prose. You are not striving for a Pulitzer. This is not a comprehensive review of the field. Simple, direct language is key, with an emphasis on omitting needless words—such verbiage is often identified by "fresh" readers of your drafts.

Sometimes these extra words come in the form of modifiers, which should be limited overall and definitely be limited to those that are clarifying scientific descriptors ("highly conserved," "strong signal," "weakly fluorescent"). Anything that is significant should have the type of significance described ("statistically," "clinically," "biologically"). The direction of regulation should be described ("up," "down"). As noted previously, an action or activity that is "affected" should have that effect described via the verb used ("inhibited," "overexpressed," "decoupled") rather than forcing the reviewer to guess (or by adding extra words to describe it).

Similarly, you might not want to explicitly describe your ideas or approach as novel or innovative: the reviewer prefers to come to this conclusion on his or her own based on your science (and might not appreciate being told by you that your work is novel and innovative, given your personal bias). Consider the reviewer to be from Missouri (the "Show Me"). You especially do not want to tell the reviewer your project is "highly innovative" or "uniquely novel." On the other hand, a newly developed tool, assay, or other resource used in the course of your research could be described as novel, if it is both new and customized to your application.

Beyond the Text

The NIH accepts the submission of videos as nontraditional application materials. However, you cannot (at the time of this writing) embed the video directly in your Research Strategy file but must submit it to the SRO of your study section after the application has been accepted and referred for review.

While you will need to review the full policy statement on videos in NIH grant applications (at the time of this writing, http://grants.nih.gov/grants/guide/notice-files/NOT-OD-12-141.html) for all the restrictions and instructions, here are the key points:

- The only acceptable content for videos is demonstrations of devices and experimental data with a temporal element, which refers to the need to show how something functions or occurs over time, or demonstrates movement or change.

- The cover letter submitted with the application must include information about the intent to submit a video; if this is not done, a video will not be accepted. Key images/"stills" and a brief description of each video must be included within the page limits of the Research Strategy.
- Multiple videos may be submitted per application, but their aggregate length must not exceed 2 minutes for single-project applications and 5 minutes for multicomponent applications.
- Post-submission videos must be embedded in.pdf files with a maximum file size of 25 MB. This material can be submitted on CD/DVD or via e-mail, and it will be uploaded to the grant folder by the SRO.
- Applications submitted with hyperlinks to videos or with videos embedded in the research strategy will be considered in violation of page limits, and the application will be withdrawn before review.

You should check for updates to this policy, as the NIH may gradually migrate toward permitting videos to be embedded within the actual application submitted. However, this will require considerable labor to monitor, so the policy of having video material vetted by the receiving SRO may be continued indefinitely.

10

Getting by with a Little Help from Your Friends

THERE IS NO need to keep the joy of preparing a grant application all to yourself. You have an exciting, compelling idea that everyone will want to read about in the literature in a few years. Your friends should be happy to read about this now and to let you know whether you have conveyed just how important and exciting your research is. More important, you do not want to surprise your Program Officer (PO) by having your application land on his or her desk without having heard from you in advance of submission.

Friends at the National Institutes of Health

Many investigators, particularly new investigators, do not realize that they can or should communicate with NIH program staff directly. In fact, not only is such interaction allowed, it is strongly encouraged. Since POs were often investigators before moving into their present positions, they remain deeply engaged with the research in their portfolio and come to look at these principal investigators (PIs) as "their investigators" (see also Chapter 3, where a goal in communicating with your assigned reviewers is to have them come to think of you as one of "their investigators").

You should contact program staff throughout the application process, starting in the planning stages. See the Appendix for links to program staff at each IC. Many Funding Opportunity Announcements (FOAs) list the PO(s) assigned to that program as the Scientific/Research Contact(s) You can also search RePORTER (see Chapters 4 and 6) to see which POs have been assigned to funded research that is similar to yours, and you can talk with mentors and colleagues for additional suggestions. Once you make contact with the right PO at one IC, if your work might be of interest to another IC (as a primary or secondary assignment), you might ask this PO for suggestions on whom to contact at the other IC(s) or identify them via the same methods.

POs vary in terms of whether they prefer to communicate via e-mail or on the phone. You should start with an e-mail and inquire as to their preference and then inquire about dates and times to talk, if they prefer telephone discussions. Please keep in mind that, in addition to working with hundreds of extramural researchers such as you, POs also serve on committees, write reports, and attend seminars and symposia, so you should not assume your PO can immediately respond or talk. If your PO of choice does not respond after a few attempts, you can look around for someone else in that IC subunit who might be appropriate or inquire one level up with the division or unit chief for referral.

Once you have connected with the best PO(s), discussions and correspondence can be wide ranging, depending on your career status and goals, research area, and any unique circumstances. You can make such communication constructive by first exploring the NIH Guide (http://grants.nih.gov/grants/guide/index.html) for funding possibilities, your target IC Web site for their research priorities, and RePORTER (http://projectreporter.nih.gov/reporter.cfm) to identify what studies are currently being funded in your area of interest.

In your initial communication, you will want to send a brief overview of your aims and approach, no more than three to four paragraphs, including the approximate annual cost and project duration. For mentored training and career development mechanisms, you will want to include the name of your mentor(s) and their funding source.

Most POs are happy to discuss research and funding opportunities, appropriate mechanisms, career development issues, and the application and peer review process. Once you begin to develop a specific application, some POs are willing to give advice on your goals, research questions, overall study design and methods, and potential collaborators; do not expect them to weigh in on methodological details or other finer points of the Approach, though. You can ask, while developing the application (versus when you are almost done), about which study sections to target (more in Chapter 3); POs attend review meetings and know the Scientific Review Officers (SROs) and the culture of the study sections that handle research in their areas.

Some etiquette tips: e-mail traffic can be very heavy for many POs, so if a few days have passed without any response, do not hesitate to send a reminder e-mail. Only "cold call" if you have a simple, straightforward question or need a quick confirmation related to an issue you have previously discussed. You could be calling 5 minutes before the PO is due at a meeting. You should not call just to chat, and all communication should be focused rather than rambling. Plan ahead about what you will say (write down your questions and discussion points, since the conversation may get you off track of your original thoughts), and of course give your PO plenty of time to read your proposal ideas. They are juggling multiple deadlines, projects, and investigators, so being respectful of their time and helping them make the most effective use of your time together will be greatly appreciated and remembered the next time you want to discuss something.

There, of course, are times that it is not useful to contact the PO, and your abstinence from doing so will likewise be appreciated. From the time you submit your application until you receive your summary statement, your PO will not be able to comment on the status of your application. If you have concerns about the study section assignment or who is on the roster, you should contact the SRO, though you can also ask your PO for advice on whether to change study sections.

Although you will be tempted to contact your PO when you see your impact score and, if applicable, percentile in eRA Commons, please wait until you have your summary statement. Except for very late in the fiscal year (see Chapter 5) or with exceptional impact scores, your PO will likely not be able to comment on your funding chances, so please do not be disappointed if this is the case; it will be the norm for the first few months of the fiscal year and often longer.

With your summary statement in hand, the discussion can cover more than "will I be funded?" You will be able to ask for guidance in responding to the critiques and revising the application, if this was your initial (A0) submission. If your PO heard the discussion of your application, he or she might be able to clarify a concern raised. Especially if your IC develops paylists without a "hard" payline, your PO may ask you how you would respond to the weaknesses cited. If your score is in the "gray zone" (near the putative payline), such a discussion will help the PO know whether he or she can recommend your application for funding; such a recommendation is more likely if the concerns raised were procedural rather than related to the underlying science or overall approach. We will cover your options upon receiving your summary statement in more detail in Chapters 11 and 13 (including an explanation of priority scores, percentiles, paylines, select pay, and success rates)—just know that your PO will play a key role.

Most POs should be able to provide some guidance on funding likelihood after the IC Council meets (see http://citfm.cit.nih.gov/ofacp/meetings. php for a complete schedule of all NIH Council meetings); IC staff and, ultimately, the IC Director decide after this meeting which applications will receive an award. How soon afterward varies depending on the status of the NIH appropriation from Congress (Chapter 5). POs are notoriously conservative in raising expectations, but even if they are "cautiously optimistic" (translation: yours is on the list of applications to be awarded but has not been signed yet—and anything could happen in strange budget times), remember that nothing is final until you have a Notice of Award.

Even after, in fact, especially after, receiving an award, you should still keep in regular contact with your PO. You will be providing progress reports annually as part of the noncompeting renewal process, but your PO will want to know about articles accepted for publication (which must also be deposited in PubMed Central, as noted in Chapter 14), patent applications filed, and new, interesting results. Your IC or the NIH may want to issue a news release for a publication resulting from your work, so be sure to inform your PO as soon as you learn a manuscript is likely to be accepted; he or she will need enough lead time to work with your university public information office and the IC communications personnel in preparing a media packet. Plus, your PO will want to brag to colleagues about your productive research as part of his or her portfolio, and your PO can give you advance notice of new initiatives being planned at the IC. POs enjoy meeting with "their investigators" at scientific conferences or workshops (assuming the NIH appropriation allows for such travel by staff), so by all means, contact yours in advance to see whether you can arrange to meet during a coffee break, meal, or poster session.

Friends outside the National Institutes of Health

The more eyes on your proposal, the better. No matter how many times you read something, you will miss omissions, mistakes, and logic gaps. You will also lose track of how you can make the narrative as easy and pleasant for the reviewer as possible, because you will reach the point that you yourself no longer want to read the document.

You might want to take a divide-and-conquer approach. Mentors, collaborators, and lab or clinic personnel would be most appropriate to comment on the overall idea and specific components of the Approach. Colleagues in your field but not your specific area of investigation will have a fresh perspective on whether your Significance and Innovation are compelling. Feedback from anyone outside your field, whether friends or professional writers ("grant writers"), can help gauge whether you have conveyed your intended message and meaning.

If you have developed the narrative in a compelling, reviewer-friendly style, reading it straight through without making corrections along the way should not be burdensome. You do not want a quick, noncritical reading of your narrative by a friend to take more than an hour. If so, the narrative style or presentation may be too complex or dense for study section reviewers as well, even those who are assigned and will take more time with the proposal. This can be a sign that you may need to better develop your ideas to the point at which you can present them clearly and concisely. Again, your goal is to make the reviewer's job as easy and pleasant as possible.

Some universities have grant development resources available to faculty and trainees. These could include workshops on grantsmanship, a repository of funded applications, grant administrators to help with the preparation of the budget, and science writer/editors to review and help revise the narrative. If you hire outside assistance, please remember the best service such individuals can provide, rather than actually helping "write" the application, is one of a naïve reviewer who can tell you what you are actually communicating, whether it is your intended message or not. In the end, though, no amount of writing or grantsmanship excellence will overcome science that is not exciting to the reviewer, so you should not turn to such services with the expectation that funding will be guaranteed (or nearly so).

11

Before and after Your Study Section Meets

ONCE YOU HAVE submitted your application, the waiting game begins, but it is not a passive period. Not by a long shot.

Before the Review

As we discussed in Chapter 10, your Program Officer (PO) will not be able to comment on your application until you have your summary statement. You might have contacted your PO if your application was not assigned to the scientific review group (SRG) you requested, but once the assignment is made, any communications with your PO should be about your next application (or a funded one) rather than the one under review.

You will have one formal opportunity to interact with the Scientific Review Officer (SRO) between the application submission and review. About 6 weeks prior to the SRG meeting, the SRO may invite all applicants to send eligible postsubmission application materials per NIH policy guidelines (most recent as of this writing at http://grants.nih.gov/grants/guide/notice-files/NOT-OD-13-030.html). If you do not receive a request from your SRO, please just remember that all postsubmission materials must be received at least 30 days prior to the scheduled study section meeting date.

For the most part, such materials are limited to address unforeseen administrative issues, such as revised budget, biographical sketches, and letters of support or collaboration due to newly awarded overlapping funding, the acquisition of equipment originally requested, losses due to a natural disaster, the tenure or other promotion of any senior/key personnel, changes in senior/key personnel (replacement or loss of an investigator since submission—but not just to add an investigator who was left off the original application), and a change of institution by the principal investigator (PI) (more on this last item in Chapter 14).

For institutional training grant applications (but not individual fellowships/F or career development/K applications), you can provide updates on any trainee's (past or current) or faculty member's graduation, employment, promotion, publication, funding, or other professional achievement. Information on new faculty members who will be involved in the training program can be provided as well.

You can also send news of and, if available, the citation for an article accepted for publication since the original submission (but not a copy of the manuscript itself).

Some funding opportunity announcements (FOAs) permit other post-submission materials, and your SRO will inform you of what is allowable and in what format the materials should be submitted. This is particularly true of Requests for Applicatiosn (RFAs) with just one submission date (or for applications in response to the last submission date), in which case late-breaking data and adjustments to the Specific Aims may be allowed—but, again, you will receive instructions from the SRO.

In general, all postsubmission materials follow the same formatting guidelines for NIH applications (font size, margins, paper size, etc.), and materials such as biographical sketches, budget information, and other information provided in the main application on specified form pages should likewise be submitted on these form pages. The number of postsubmission material pages depends on the length of the research strategy of the original application (1 page of postsubmission material for a Research Strategy that is less than 12 pages, 2 pages for 12 pages, and 3 pages for more than 12 pages). Everything is submitted as a PDF attachment.

Videos can submitted so long as you indicate in the cover letter (required, not optional) that a video will be sent after the application is referred for review and that you incorporate in the Research Strategy itself (as submitted) any still images and description needed to convey the content of the video, since reviewers will not be obligated to view it (see also Chapter 9). Currently, the "only acceptable content for videos is demonstrations of devices and experimental data with a temporal element, which refers to the need to show how something functions or occurs over time, or demonstrates movement or change." The policy for video submissions will likely evolve over time from the original notice (http://grants.nih.gov/grants/guide/notice-files/NOT-OD-12-141.html).

One final note: your Authorized Organization Representative (AOR), usually the director of your sponsored programs or research office, must concur with any postapplication submission. You cannot merely carbon copy (cc) the AOR. Either your AOR must submit the materials to the SRO, or you must receive from your AOR a message concurring with the materials, which you then forward to the SRO. The SRO, not you, uploads these materials to your application in eRA Commons.

Review Week

You may as well resign yourself to hitting refresh on your eRA Commons account every 10 minutes starting the day after your study section meets. Your score may not be posted for a few days, though, depending on the number of applications submitted and discussed. Try not to read anything good or bad into any delay, real or perceived.

When that climatic moment finally occurs, your score may be posted without a percentile—and not all applications receive a percentile.

For more than half of you, this moment will be a crushing disappointment. Either your application will be listed as "Not Discussed," or your score will clearly not be in funding range. Chapter 13 gives suggestions on what to do next.

Please remember that any score, even one not likely to result in funding is useful: you will receive reviewer comments and a summary of the group discussion to guide the development of your next application, plus whatever insight your PO can offer based on what he or she might have heard during the study section meeting. Depending on your career status, you will have a score to wave at higher-ups who are making decisions about hiring, renewing contracts, promotions, and institutional bridge funding.

After the Review

Once you have your summary statement, you can contact your PO. Whether your PO will be able to tell you much about your chances for funding depends mainly on the status of the federal budget (Chapter 5), both in terms of timing and dollar amounts. Please be aware that, especially if your IC has not posted any paylines (interim or final), your PO will be conservative in giving any encouragement unless you received a 10 (and in some cases, even this is not a guarantee!). Also, if your PO says he or she does not know the payline, he or she does not—they are not withholding information, they truly do not know.

If your score is in the "gray zone" with regard to funding chances, you may want to start working on your revised application, assuming you can readily address the concerns raised and submit a strong A1 quickly. The A0 remains under consideration even after the A1 is reviewed and scored, which, yes, can occur before the outcome of the A0 is known; also, you do not lose a review cycle in case your A0 is not selected for funding. In the eRA Commons account shown in Figure 11.1, both the A0 and the A1 of the National Institute of Diabetes and Digestive and Kidney Diseases (DK) R21 remain under active consideration, whereas an old R21 application submitted 2 years prior has been administratively withdrawn (no longer under consideration for funding) by the National Institute of Alcohol Abuse and Alcoholism (AA).

You should always continue your research after the application is submitted with an eye toward possible resubmission, so that you are ready to do so as needed. You generally cannot afford to lose more than one cycle, or your significance, innovation, and impact may suffer as the field moves forward. Chapter 13 discusses resubmission strategies in more detail, including deciding whether to wait—the goal is always to submit the strongest possible application.

If you are a new or early-stage investigator (ESI) applicant and the application was in response to an FOA with standard receipt dates, you should quickly decide whether to take advantage of the rapid resubmission (about 6 weeks after you receive your summary statement). You should

1R21DK102090-01	GRANT11432053	Analysis of Idiopathic Pancreatitis in the NAPS2 GWAS	WHITCOMB, DAVID CLEMENT	Submission Complete	Pending IRG Review	07/03/2013	Transmittal Sheet
1R21DK098560-01A1	GRANT11356482	Evaluation of Pain in Chronic Pancreatitis using the NAPS2 cohorts	WHITCOMB, DAVID CLEMENT	Submission Complete	Pending Council Review	06/05/2013	JIT | Transmittal Sheet
1R21DK098560-01	GRANT11164137	Evaluation of Pain in Chronic Pancreatitis using the NAPS2 cohorts	WHITCOMB, DAVID CLEMENT	Submission Complete	Council review completed	02/14/2013	JIT | Transmittal Sheet
1R21AA017283-01	GRANT00206308	Exploratory Program in Complex Genetics of Alcohol and Pancreatitis	WHITCOMB, DAVID C	Submission Complete	Administratively Withdrawn by IC	11/08/2011	Transmittal Sheet

FIGURE 11.1 Screen shot of eRA Commons account showing application status, including A0 and A1 versions of the same application that are simultaneously under consideration for funding.

consider this route if the concerns are straightforward and easily addressable and do not require additional preliminary data that you do not have on hand (more on this in Chapter 13).

In addition to discussing funding likelihood and when this might be known, you can talk with your PO about the topics to be detailed in Chapter 13: whether to resubmit (if your score is for an A0 or new submission), strategies for the resubmission if you can, and strategies for repurposing the application if not.

Council Meeting

If your IC is one of the few that posts interim paylines and your score falls within them, please remember that you still need to wait for Council to provide the second level of review. Many PIs do not realize that Council members are assigned applications being considered by the IC for funding and that they do review the summary statement and sometimes the application itself. You can find the operating procedures for the Advisory Council of your IC(s) on their Web site (see Appendix).

Council receives electronic access to summary statements and applications under consideration for funding (all mechanisms except individual fellowships) about 6 to 8 weeks in advance of their meeting. Council members do not have access to summary statements or applications from their own institution. Council members with questions or who need additional information about a specific application as part of their second-level review will contact the assigned PO.

Some R01 and R21 applications receive Council approval for funding consideration through an online process of either early or expedited concurrence. If your eRA Commons status changes to "Council review completed" before the published Council meeting date, your application has likely been approved for consideration through one of these electronic processes.

Council members can tap individual applications for discussion at the Council meeting due to a policy issue, budget questions, or concerns about the SRG discussion or recommendations—or simply because the Council member finds the research of particular interest or importance to the IC. A Council member can also suggest that an application be considered for pay by exception or select pay (no additional review needed). On the other hand, a Council member can disagree with the SRG recommendation and recommend that an application not be considered for funding for reasons other than scientific merit, such as significant levels of other funding to the PI or lack of priority to the IC, especially if the same or similar research is currently being funded.

Unlike the SRG reviewers, Council members are not just judging the scientific merit but also whether the research fits the mission and meets the current priorities of the IC. They also check applications for administrative concerns raised at review (human subjects, vertebrate animals, resource sharing, biohazards). They consider MERIT award (R37) nominations and extensions, appeal letters from PIs who disagree with their SRG review, and applications from foreign institutions that meet the criteria for funding.

As with study section reviewers, Council members are prohibited from disclosing any information related to an application or its review by either the SRG or Council. All materials distributed at a Council meeting are collected and destroyed. The NIH takes the protection of the confidentiality of all review proceedings very seriously.

Council also hears presentations about research initiatives the IC would like to undertake and votes on these as "cleared concepts," which you should keep track of so as to anticipate upcoming FOAs of particular relevance to your area of research. Some ICs highlight their cleared concepts on a specific Web site (e.g., NCI, ; NIAID, http://www.niaid.nih.gov/researchfunding/council/concepts/pages/default.aspx, and NIMH, http://www.nimh.nih.gov/about/advisory-boards-and-groups/namhc/namhc-concept-clearances.shtml), while for most, you would need to review the latest Council minutes (see Appendix for Websites).

Appeals

Even if your every instinct screams "appeal" after you have read the summary statement, you should not use this term—as in wanting to make a formal appeal—with your PO but instead discuss your concerns informally first. Formally appealing an SRG recommendation is usually not the best option.

First, there is the time lost. Unless both the CSR and IC staff determine that your review was clearly flawed based on objective scientific grounds (see the full policy at the time of this writing at http://grants.nih.gov/grants/guide/notice-files/NOT-OD-11-064.html), your appeal will go to the next Council meeting for consideration. If Council denies your appeal, you must wait until the next funding cycle to resubmit your A1 (if the A0 was appealed). If Council approves your appeal, your application cannot be changed but will be re-reviewed as originally submitted at the next review cycle. Then you must wait for another Council meeting for the second-level review and so on. If your appealed application was an A0 and it still does not achieve a fundable score, you are now multiple cycles (a year or more) behind with the A1 submission.

Second, there is your potentially damaged relationship with the SRG, which could be very important, depending on how flexible you are in sending applications to other study sections in the future; if these are your best reviewers, you want to stay on good terms with them. If your appeal is accepted, your application will be sent unchanged to reviewers who now know you disagreed with their prior review so much that you convinced Council it was in error. This is not the mindset you want your go-to reviewers to be in.

If your summary statement includes criticisms that unequivocally affected your score (to the point that your outcome would have been different) and can clearly and objectively be linked to scientific error (versus a difference of opinion or interpretation), then you can prepare a few bullets addressing this error for your PO to consider for guidance on whether you should appeal.

Remember, the error must be so large as to significantly affect your final impact score (not just annoy you), and this is quite difficult to gauge, since you cannot use the individual criterion scores of each reviewer to calculate the SRG-assigned priority score. A misunderstanding that would not have likely added 10 or more points to your score is not worth a fight, though it must be addressed in the resubmission (if eligible), and the SRO should be told which reviewer(s) made the error, so they are not reassigned.

If your PO agrees that your first review was scientifically flawed and that you should appeal, you will still resubmit the exact same application (no revisions or new data) for review by a new set of SRG members, though you do not have to wait for Council action in the meantime. If the score comes back roughly the same, as noted earlier, you will have lost considerable time in moving on with a better application.

Administrative Review and Award Processing

Once Council has approved your application for consideration for funding, whether before electronically or at the Council meeting itself, it can be administratively reviewed for compliance with NIH policies and adjustments in the amounts and terms of the award. Processing of an R01 award can begin early if you are at a US institution and your score is at or better than the current or anticipated payline.

An assigned overall impact score of 40 or less will generate an automatic JIT request in eRA Commons, but you should wait until you receive a request from your PO or Grant Management Specialist (GMS) before preparing this information. JIT requests are sometimes issued before final funding decisions have been made so that those selected for awards can be quickly processed; at some ICs, only those applications selected for an award undergo administrative review.

When you receive a JIT request from your IC, if you are unsure, you can ask your PO as to whether an award is just being considered or if your application is being processed for an award.

You may be interested to learn Congress receives a list of all awards to be made by an IC at least 45 hours prior to Notices of Award (NoAs) being issued (72 hours in advance for awards exceeding $1 million, with notification sent to the White House as well). Your Congressional delegation will learn of all awards made to your institution—and hopefully will recognize the economic value of such funding in his or her District. As we mention in Chapter 5, you can help remind your elected delegation of the importance of supporting the NIH budget not only to advance biomedical research and improve public health but also to strengthen the local economy.

Your NoA lists the approved budget for each year (direct, indirect, total costs) and whether the award is eligible for Streamlined Noncompeting Award Process (SNAP), in which case an electronic Research Performance Progress Report (RPPR) is submitted electronically through eRA Commons. The NoA includes information on the requirement for the PI to comply with the NIH Public Access Policy in order to secure noncompeting renewal funds in subsequent years. Your institution indicates its acceptance of the award, including its Terms and Conditions, when it starts drawing on the funds. And you are an NIH-funded investigator. Simple.

12

Is the Check in the Mail?

AS WE EXPLAIN in Chapter 5, unless your score is truly exceptional, the status of the federal budget will determine whether your Program Officer (PO) will know the funding likelihood of your application. Chapter 3 discusses how the review is conducted and how overall impact/priority scores and percentiles are determined. Chapter 2 includes details for some Institutes and Centers (ICs) as to how they arrive at paylines or paylists to guide funding decisions. We will briefly review these concepts again here, to pull them together with success rates as well.

Reading the Numbers

Your score is based solely on the scientific merit of your application and overall impact of your proposed research as rated by the entire study section (never calculated from the individual criterion scores listed on your summary statement).

Your percentile is linked with your study section, not your IC (see Chapter 3 for details on how this is calculated).

The payline is set by your IC as a funding threshold or range and can be based on either score or percentile (see Chapter 2 for some IC-specific details). Generally, the payline does not take into account the application type (new or Type 1 versus competing renewal or Type 2) or status (initial or Ao versus resubmitted or A1). Some ICs, such as the National Heart, Lung and Blood Institute (NHLBI), http://www.nhlbi.nih.gov/funding/policies/archive/operguid11.htm, have in the past set graduated paylines by amendment type (i.e., a higher payline for Ao than for A1), but this stopped at the

NHLBI after the A2 submission was discontinued. In addition, some ICs try to help new or ESI applicants seeking to renew (Type 2) their first R01 award.

The success rate (percentage of applications reviewed that are funded) is distinct from both your application percentile and the IC's payline (Chapter 6 explains where to find these data). Success rates are typically higher than the payline or paylist percentile range, in part because applications for which both A0 and A1 versions have been reviewed in the same year (e.g., February and November) are only counted once. In addition, success rate does vary not only by activity code but also by application type and amendment status.

Thus, an application that receives, for example, an overall impact score of 12 that ranks in the 5th percentile would be within the IC payline and receive an award. However, the success rate attributed to the application category for this award would depend on its submission type and status:

- Type 1 A0: 8.6%
- Type 1 A1: 37.2%
- Type 2 A0: 28.4%
- Type 2 A1: 49.7%

In other words, almost half of all revised submissions of competing renewals received a score in the percentile range required to obtain an award, whereas fewer than one in ten new initial applications fared as well (see Chapter 6 for details on how to find these data, which are for FY12). This is not surprising since the pool of competing renewal applications is smaller, and most PIs do not submit a competing renewal if they know they have not been sufficiently productive in terms of publications on research completed during the last award period.

Similarly, for the most part, A1 applications are submitted by PIs who received a score for their A0 application, again resulting in a smaller applicant pool with subsequently higher success rate. The mere process of submitting an A1 just to submit one does not mean you will have a higher success rate if, for example, your A0 application was not scored or if the reviewers did not feel the work itself was significant (a difficult concern to adequately address, as discussed in Chapter 13).

When Will You Know Whether Your Score Is "Fundable"

You will likely know whether your score is "fundable" immediately when your eRA Commons account is updated: about half of all applications will receive an ND designation (Not Discussed, also referred to as triaged or streamlined), though this varies by IC. The research project grant (RPG) data shown in Table 12.1 are provided by IC rather than SRG, but this gives you a comparison of scoring of applications of scientific interest to the ICs; some ICs, such as National Library of Medicine, review most applications assigned internally, so these data reflect a mix of Center for Scientific Review (CSR) and IC study section practices. The Career Development data reflect discussion trends for both the SRG (since these applications are reviewed by IC-specific rather than CSR study sections) and the IC; these data are for all K mechanisms combined, and not all ICs participate in all the mechanisms.

If you do have a score, you can be hopeful if it is below 20 or has a single-digit percentile ranking. Your PO should be able to confirm your hope, perhaps with a statement of being "cautiously optimistic," though you should still wait to contact him or her until you the summary statement is posted to your eRA Commons account.

For most applications, whether your score predicts your funding likelihood depends on the time of year (see Chapter 5). If the fiscal year appropriation is known, those ICs that publish numeric paylines should have these available; if the federal government is operating under a continuing resolution, the ICs may have interim paylines, with the final numbers not available until the federal budget is established. For those ICs that do not publish their paylines, you will need to check with your PO—again, waiting until you have your summary statement (more on this in Chapter 11).

The question to ask at this point is not whether you will be funded but whether your application is under consideration for funding. Particularly with the degree of federal budget dysfunction in recent years (see Chapter 5), your PO will likely not know about whether your application will receive an award, if it is not clearly within the typical funding range, until late in the fiscal year.

As a reminder (from Chapter 2), at some ICs, such as the National Institute of Allergy and Infectious Diseases, the payline is "hard" and based strictly on score or percentile, while at others, such as National Institute of General Medical Sciences, all applications within a certain score or percentile range are discussed at the Branch or Division level to select applications to recommend to the Director for funding (https://loop.nigms.nih.gov/index.php/2011/01/28/the-funding-decision-process/). In Figure 12.1, we present summary funding trend data for FY12 based on the ICs for which these data were available; Chapter 2 provides these data by individual IC (where available). You can see what percentage of applications that were scored at a given percentile were likely to receive awards.

Table 12.1 Number and Percentage of Research Project and Career Development Applications Discussed at each IC

IC	Research Grant Applications			Career Development Applications		
	No. Discussed	No. of Applications	% Discussed	No. Discussed	No. of Applications	% Discussed
NCI	5,999	10,796	55.6	222	476	46.6
NHLBI	4,076	7,079	57.6	304	461	65.9
NIDCR	638	1,012	63.0	37	38	97.4
NIDDK	2,782	4,469	62.3	357	362	98.6
NINDS	2,748	4,899	56.2	123	198	62.1
NIAID	4,270	7,621	56.0	128	219	58.4
NIGMS	3,213	5,639	57.0	95	194	49.0
NICHD	2,571	4,745	54.2	189	251	75.3
NEI	789	1,372	57.5	30	30	100.0
NIEHS	767	1,659	46.2	36	41	87.8
NIA	1,552	2,830	54.8	164	175	93.7
NIAMS	1,169	2,146	54.5	98	112	87.5
NIDCD	496	932	53.2	21	45	46.7
NIMH	2,053	3,757	54.6	192	264	72.7
NIDA	1,432	2,472	57.9	89	147	60.5

NIAAA	676	58.8	1,150	61	73	83.6
NINR	452	54.7	827	40	43	93.0
NHGRI	369	60.1	614	12	13	92.3
NIBIB	1,058	50.4	2,101	38	63	55.9
NCCAM	300	44.2	678	29	35	82.9
NIMHD	190	48.1	395	2	2	100
FIC	163	68.5	238	15	20	75.0
NLM	207	86.3	240	23	23	100
OD	552	20.8	2,651	23	24	95.8
NCATS	171	74.3	230	15	15	100
NIH	38,693	54.9%	70,542	2,313	3,324	69.6%

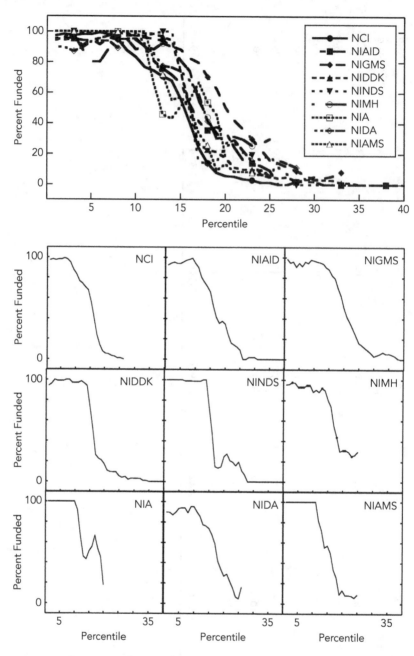

FIGURE 12.1 Percentage of R01 applications funded at each percentile in FY12 at 9 ICs.

Your PO is the one to advocate for your application for select pay or pay by exception or at paylist meetings, for those ICs that use this process. In some cases, your PO will request a one-page rebuttal to the major concerns raised by reviewers—concerns generally with methodological details rather than the underlying science or assumptions. If you have exciting new data, a recent presentation at a scientific meeting, or a manuscript under review, or, even better, accepted for publication, these would all be important updates to pass along to your PO.

Also, if your score is close and the concerns focus on one Aim, you can indicate to your PO whether you can reduce the scope of work to eliminate the weak aim and focus on work for which the reviewers showed enthusiasm, with the idea that your PO might be able to advocate for either a shortened R01 or a 1-year R56 (see Chapter 7). There is little you can do, as your PO must initiate any of these actions, but you should be aware of some of these alternative (albeit lesser) pathways to funding.

No matter your score, please be patient and realize that your PO is not hiding secret information from you. Although you want (and possibly, for career reasons, need) a more definitive response sooner, their conservative judgment of your chances of funding or a response that no information is available about the payline/paylist does in fact reflect how much (or little) they know. If you let them know about any extenuating circumstances such as a tenure decision (including relevant time-sensitive dates), they will know to be in touch when information does come available, though not necessarily by the time you would like (or need) an answer. Please realize that your PO will have scores of PIs asking the same question, feeling the same career stress.

Once again, if the federal budget has not been set, POs will not know about paylines/paylists, nor will the Director of the IC.

The POs want to have good news—any news—for you, so if you have asked once and been told they do not have any information about the status of your application, politely ask them to let you know when they do, and trust that they will be in touch when they have updated information to pass along. Of course, requests for advice about revising the application, other funding opportunities, developing a new application, and so on (see Chapter 11) would certainly be appropriate during the waiting period.

Mostly, though, you will just have to hurry up and wait.

13

The Check Is Not
in the Mail . . .

SO YOUR APPLICATION was not discussed, or it received a score that will not make the paylist. What next?

If this was your first submission (A0), you have one opportunity to revise and resubmit an amended (A1) application. A significant uproar greeted the change in NIH policy regarding the number of resubmissions, from two down to one, and arguments continue in favor of restoring the second resubmission (the A2) or treating every application as new. However, it appears likely that the NIH will stick with the two-submission policy (A0, A1) for the foreseeable future (see Rock Talk for a recap, http://nexus.od.nih.gov/all/2012/11/28/the-a2-resubmission-policy-continues-a-closer-look-at-recent-data/). Their goal is to fund the best science faster, and each submission adds months and often years to the delay between the idea being formulated and funding being achieved. Fewer chances to submit applications that are not likely to receive awards also reduces reviewer burden (remember, this is a community service).

If you are a new or early-stage investigator (ESI) applicant who submitted an A0 to an R01 funding opportunity announcement (FOA) with standard receipt dates (February, June, October), you might be able to take advantage of rapid resubmission to avoid losing a cycle (see also Chapters 2 and 11). NIH policy (at the time of this writing, http://grants.nih.gov/grants/guide/notice-files/NOT-OD-11-057.html) permits new and ESI applicants to submit their A1 applications about 6 weeks after receipt of their summary statement (i.e., April, August, and December 10). Whether you should take advantage of this opportunity will depend on the concerns raised in the summary statement and progress made on your research since the A0 was submitted.

If this was an A0 that was not discussed or that received a relatively poor score, you will need to decide whether to resubmit at all or to instead develop a new application that is substantially changed from the unsuccessful A0. Applications that have not been discussed are difficult to revise and resubmit, since you do not have input from the entire study section on the strengths and weaknesses of your project. Once, a reviewer decides an application is not competitive and should not be discussed, they may not list all their concerns. However, if each of the reviewers raised the same addressable points in the summary statement and none had major concerns with the significance of the research proposed, you might consider an A1; although relatively rare, it is possible to go from unscored to funded with an A1.

At the same time, you should not assume your A1 will receive a better score than the A0, even if you address all the concerns. If the reviewers were not especially enthusiastic about the significance of the work, the score might well stay about the same, and a previously scored application could be not discussed as an A1, especially if one or more new reviewers have different concerns.

If your second submission (A1) is not discussed or is not scored competitively, you will need to decide whether to pursue the same project with a different funding mechanism (e.g., downsizing from an R01 to an R21) or to substantially revise and update the research for a new (A0) application.

We explain in Chapter 11 why appeals are generally not a good idea and suggest better strategies for working with your Program Officer (PO) to address reviewer concerns that are not scientifically valid (as confirmed by others, not just your opinion).

No matter what, this is always a good time to consider your long-term funding strategy as well (discussed at the end of the chapter).

Resubmission

As discussed in Chapter 11, you may have already started updating your A0 application while waiting for your review, in preparation for a potential resubmission (please remember when completing the SF424 electronic application that the A1 application is formally called a "resubmission," not a "revision," which refers to a Type 3 application for a competitive supplement). You may want to start integrating new findings relevant to your proposal from your own lab or data reported in the literature as they become available rather than wait until you learn the outcome of your review. Even if your A0 is funded, the exercise will help you reframe some experiments that may need to be revised based on the new data. If the review of your Ao does not result in funding and does not suggest the need to abandon this proposal, you will have a head start on the amended application.

As noted in Chapter 10, you will want to talk with your PO about your summary statement and obtain insight as to how the discussion went—especially what was said or communicated via tone and body language that might not have come across in the summary statement. This is particularly important if the Resume and Summary of Discussion at the start of the summary statement includes such phrases as "after much discussion" or "reviewers could not agree" or "some reviewers felt." Sometimes, too, the PO remembers a point that the Scientific Review Officer (SRO) did not include in the Summary of Discussion; if your PO passes along such observations, you would consider these points when revising the text but not directly address them in the Introduction). Even if the Summary of Discussion paragraph is straightforward, your PO will likely have attended other meetings of this study section and will know their habits and preferences and how to read between the lines. Your PO's experience and input will be important in deciding how and how much to revise the proposal.

We discuss in Chapter 8 strategies for preparing a reasoned, helpful Introduction to the Revised Application in which you address concerns raised in the discussion of your Ao application and summarize major improvements and additions to the A1 revision. Here, we must reiterate that you should not try to turn this into a debate and should not include any subjective or judgmental language. If need be, write a couple of drafts telling the reviewers what you really think and keep shredding these until you get closer to an objective response. Be sure to have someone outside your research read your Introduction to gauge the tone and responsiveness. Remember, it is not about you—it is all about the reviewers.

You will want to draft the Introduction before starting on your revisions, to organize the reviewer concerns in your mind in a structural (rather than emotion-laden) manner, and then go back to revise and refine the Introduction once you are done developing your revised Specific Aims and Research Strategy.

Once you have put your initial visceral response behind you, you will be able to gauge which of the weaknesses flagged are valid and capable of being addressed versus which suggestions are untenable and modify your approach accordingly. If your proposal has been labeled "overly ambitious," you will need to scale back the project. The message of proposing to do too much is that you are not sufficiently experienced to anticipate the workload involved, the potential (likely) setbacks that will occur along the way, and the time needed to complete the experiments and analyses required (e.g., multiple replications at the bench, breeding sufficient animals with the right genotype, accruing patients in the clinic, etc.). Here, your mentors and colleagues will play an important role as your sounding board in reframing work labeled "overly ambitious."

If your project is large because you need to complete certain experiments before moving on to a second phase of the work, you might consider splitting off one or two of your aims into an R21 or R03 application (see below under "Repurposing Your Application"), assuming your current submission was an R01. You can wait on the rest of the work until it can be submitted as either a delayed A1 or a new A0 that incorporates the results of the R21 or R03 secured separately.

In revising your proposal, you will need to address concerns raised in the Resume and Summary of Discussion, paying attention to any details in the individual critiques related to these concerns. Easily addressable concerns include the following:

- Lack of preliminary data (assuming you have kept busy in the meantime)
- Lack of innovation (you should be able to rework and improve your message here—it is the toughest review criterion for reviewers)
- Lack of details on the experimental design, including potential pitfalls and alternative approaches (in addition to filling in details, you want to be sure to convey you will understand how to interpret the data, even if they are negative or not what you expect)

For other mechanisms, such as career development and program grants, you should be able to address alack of institutional support in a straightforward fashion, assuming you have the support. Overcoming lack of productivity (especially for competing renewals) will require additional publications, which may or may not be feasible in a timely fashion.

You may also be wise to seek out new collaborators, especially if the reviewers specifically flagged the absence of appropriate expertise in a certain aspect of the work. The discussions involved in finding and establishing an appropriate collaboration could well lead to good insight into how best to address your scientific question and an innovative approach that would not have occurred to you without such input. Even if the added relationship is one of consulting rather than collaborating, the fresh perspective will be useful. Just be sure the letters written by your collaborators and consultants reflect their understanding of and enthusiasm for your project—ditto for the personal statement on their Biosketch. You do not want reviewers left feeling you have added a name rather than a team member.

However, concerns about low significance or modest impact of the research (even if completed as proposed), if raised by more than one reviewer, can be difficult to overcome unless the writing style was also flagged as a weakness. In the latter case, you may simply not have conveyed the true significance. This is where input from your PO and colleagues can help you distinguish a fixable marketing message from science that will never excite the reviewers, no matter how well written.

As you revise the application, you need to convey to reviewers what text has been substantially changed without making the narrative difficult to read. As suggested in Chapter 9, this might best be accomplished through indenting, vertical lines in the margin, or a change in font (e.g., if you use Arial for your main text, use a serif font such as Palatino or Georgia for revised text). You do not want to use bold, italic, underlined, shaded, or colored typeface, any of which could make the text more difficult to read (and confusing, if similar stylistic emphasis is used to designate major headings, key concepts, or callouts).

Timing

A final practical point: timing. You must submit your A1 application within 37 months of the A0. You should not be approaching this deadline for a resubmission, however, since the science will likely have progressed to the point that a modest revision of your original study is no longer of high impact. If the field has not progressed, your project was probably not sufficiently significant to start with (hence the lack of funding). However, as more and more time passes between the original submission and the revised application, consider whether it would be better to rework your ideas into a new A0 application.

If you have submitted one or two of your original R01 aims as a new R21 or R03 application as suggested earlier, even if you still have time to submit A1, new data generated and reports in the literature since the A0 submission could well support the development of a new R01 A0 application. You can discuss this with your PO, should the need arise; you will still want to take care that any new A0 aims do not overlap with those of the prior A0.

As discussed earlier in this chapter, for those new and ESI applicants who can take advantage of the rapid resubmission, doing so is not always advantageous. The theoretical benefit is to get funded sooner. However, if your rapid resubmission is for the April 10 receipt date, federal budget delays (see Chapter 5) may similarly push back any decision about your A1 from December until the next spring, or about the same time period as A1 applications submitted in July. So, rather than hurry to take advantage of rapid resubmission in Cycle 1 (April 10), you may be better off waiting until Cycle 2 (July 5 receipt date), if waiting would allow you to prepare a stronger, more polished revised application and to publish additional preliminary data.

Actually, the same advice on timing would apply to anyone who is deciding whether to rush in an A1 for any mechanism for the March receipt dates: there probably is no need, if your sole rationale is an earlier start date, given the history of federal budget delays. If you need to submit the application sooner to support a tenure decision, however, then those time pressures could have priority over waiting to strengthen the application.

Now, if your score is in the gray zone, you do not need or want to wait until the fate of the A0 is decided before submitting your A1 application, assuming you have a strong proposal ready (more on this in Chapter 11). You may not know the fate of the A0 until September—the very end—of the fiscal year in which it is being considered, which means you would not submit the A1 until November and not know about A1 funding until the following summer—a long time to wait, especially if your A0 had been submitted in February, more than 2 years prior.

Your A0 remains under consideration for funding even after the A1 is submitted and reviewed. You run the risk of your score going up rather than down (or, worse, having your A1 triaged), but this is a calculated risk with any resubmission, and the A0 is not necessarily discounted in that case, if the fiscal year in which it was submitted has not ended.

The bottom line, though, is that you should not submit an A1 until you have the strongest possible application.

Study Section: Should I Stay or Should I Go?

In almost all cases, you will want to stick with your original study section. If the overall impact score and individual criterion scores were good, one or more of the reviewers might have felt your application was "one of their applications" and in turn be surprised (and unhappy) to learn you were not funded, which could in turn motivate their heightened advocacy for your A1 application.

You will most likely get a mix of repeat and new reviewers for your A1 application. This is good if you have an enthusiastic reviewer from the prior meeting, but the new reviewers could be part of the reason addressing all the summary statement concerns does not always translate into a better score. The new reviewers might have different concerns than the prior reviewers, particularly if one or more was not a member of the study section or at the meeting when your A0 application was reviewed. The reassigned reviewers might find new problems in the updated proposal. As we mentioned earlier, a scored A0 application could be Not Discussed as an A1.

Despite these caveats, again, generally you are best off sticking with the original study section that reviewed your A0 proposal, especially if you think you will go back to this Scientific Review Group (SRG) again with future applications.

On rare occasions, your applications (A0 and A1) might straddle a change in SRGs that dissolves or merges your A0 study section with another. In this case, you would want to work with your PO to decide whether to follow members of the original SRG or to select an entirely new study section altogether based on the sort of research we describe in Chapter 3.

Also on rare occasions, you may feel the review was so inadequate or so unenthusiastic that you need to change study sections. Before doing so, however, be sure to get input and advice from your PO and senior colleagues. An outside perspective will help you decide whether the problem lies with the reviewers or the proposal.

You will need an objective reason in your cover letter to request the change, which should be worded in positive terms. You should list the expertise needed to review your proposal (not the names of reviewers though) and note that based on your examination of regular SRG member publications (and, of course, be sure to do this), those in the newly requested study section appear likely to be more knowledgeable about your work than those on the original study section.

Repurposing Your Application

For applications not funded as an A1 (or not discussed as an A0), you have a few options for the project as submitted. If you are exceedingly fortunate, your application might be appropriate for a Request for Application (RFA), allowing you to use the last summary statement to strengthen the proposal (but not write an Introduction in response to the prior review, of course). Similarly, any application submitted to an RFA that is not funded will be considered "new" upon subsequent submission to a Program Announcement whether a PA, PAR, or PAS, so this is another opportunity, albeit limited to special cases, to get three submissions for essentially the same proposal.

More often, though, you will need to make significant modifications to an unfunded application. If this was an R01, you could submit a smaller piece of the proposal as an R21 or R03, if your target Institute or Center (IC) participates in the parent announcement or has an FOA appropriate to your science for one of these activity codes. The R21 would allow you to obtain more preliminary data or even run a pilot clinical trial, whereas the R03 would be more appropriate for refining an animal model, experimental approach, or other well-defined bit of work toward developing a key research resource or pilot data for your main research program.

If your A1 was an unfunded K mechanism application, you might be able to convert the research plan into any of these mechanisms, though most likely the R21, unless you have sufficient preliminary data and publications to compete for R01 funding. On the other hand, the ICs generally prefer that new investigator and ESI applicants not use the R21 as a "starter grant," since this activity code has a limited budget and time frame, cannot be renewed, and can have paylines similar to or worse than R01s. However, you might not yet be competitive for an R01, depending on your publications and independence as a researcher, so you should consult with your PO and mentors for the best strategy given your individual situation.

Long-Term Strategy

At any point in your grant-seeking activities, but especially when faced with an unfunded A1, it is good to consider your overall long-term strategy for funding. Ideally, your research program includes independent parallel work that will be of interest to different SRGs and ICs. Ideally, you could target both major ICs and those with fewer applications and better success rates, such as submitting parallel applications to the National Cancer Institute (NCI) and the National Institute of Dental and Craniofacial Research (NIDCR) to study different aspects of head and neck cancer and, perhaps, the National Institute of Allergy and Infectious Diseases (NIAID) to study human papillomavirus in the context of head and neck cancer. Similarly, when branching out of your initial area of focus, or when considering a new direction to take, you should consider how tweaking the research might make it appealing to different SRGs, so the same group of regular study section members are not looking at another of your applications every cycle.

Consider too how opportunities at other federal agencies (e.g., National Science Foundation, Department of Defense, Department of Energy, Agency for Healthcare Research and Quality, etc.) and professional societies or foundations in your field might guide your decisions. The same basic principles discussed throughout this book apply to other possible sponsors: get to know those in charge of the program and those who will review your application and ensure that your proposal clearly conveys exciting work that will have significant impact and meet the needs and priorities of the sponsor (with any grant-seeking effort, it is largely about the reviewers and the sponsor, not you).

14

The Check Is
in the Mail, but . . .

OH, HAPPY DAY—you have received your Notice of Award (NoA)!—except...

As a quick general statement, we will cover here a few common questions among new grantees, but you should check the latest NIH Grants Policy Statement (http://grants1.nih.gov/grants/policy/policy.htm) for guidelines on administering your award and refer specific questions about your award to your assigned Grant Management Specialist (GMS). The GMS is there to help and is happy to do so—you should not feel as though asking questions might set off red flags that could threaten your award.

Downsized

Sometimes your summary statement will indicate a recommendation by the Scientific Review Officer (SRO) (based on the scientific review group [SRG] discussion) to reduce the budget by a module or a specific funding item (for detailed budgets), though you can try to defend your original budget with sound justification. However, even if your SRG was happy with the budget as submitted, Council might have recommended a reduction, or your Institute or Center (IC) may need to reduce the award amount or duration due to budgetary constraints on their end to accommodate as many awards as possible.

In addition to trimming the budget, many ICs will often shorten a 5-year R01 to 4 years unless the principal investigator (PI) is a new or early-stage investigator (ESI) or the work clearly requires the full project period (e.g., clinical trial). This is in part due to budget realities and in part due to the Congressional mandate that the average length of an NIH award be 4 years (more difficult for ICs that do not fund many R03 or R21 applications, which would otherwise help offset the longer R01 awards).

On top of IC reductions to the recommended budget, if the NIH is operating under a continuing resolution (see Chapter 5), the award will be cut by the amount set by NIH fiscal policy for operations under the Continuing Resolution; these cuts are generally restored, at least in part, once the NIH receives its final appropriation, assuming the final appropriation does not represent a cut from the prior fiscal year.

When significant political issues are pending that could affect the federal budget, such as a debt ceiling negotiation or an upcoming election, award cuts during the CR may be larger in anticipation of extended budget delays and potentially larger reductions in the NIH appropriation. With the federal sequestration in 2013, for example, ICs were routinely cutting awards by 25% and in some cases providing only 6 months of noncompeting renewal funds, pending the outcome of the final federal budget.

Please note that, for just this reason, the award amounts listed for each year in your NoA are not guaranteed: your subsequent project years could and likely will be subjected to reductions, either temporary or permanent, so you should take care to plan accordingly when making expenditures.

Occasionally, the PIs of applications with scores in the gray zone are offered a compromise, such as a shorter, smaller award. This can be a difficult compromise to assess, especially if an A1 has been submitted that might receive a better, more clearly fundable score. Generally, though, it is best to accept the lesser award to secure guaranteed funding sooner.

Change of Institution

If you have accepted or will soon accept an appointment at a different university or other institution eligible to accept your award (not always the case, such as if you move from an institution that qualifies for R15 funding to one that does not), you will want to communicate with your Program Officer (PO) about the impending change as soon as you know you are relocating (at the time of writing, http://grants.nih.gov/grants/policy/ nihgps_2012/nihgps_ch8.htm#_Toc271264936). The process of transferring your grant award(s) can take months. You must complete an electronic Type 7 application (at the time of writing, http://grants.nih.gov/ grants/guide/pa-files/PA-12-270.html), and your original institution (the grantee on your NoA) must relinquish the award to your new institution. You will need to demonstrate that your research can be performed at the new institution, as evidenced by appropriate support, facilities, equipment, and, if applicable, mentorship. Transferring awards is usually not blocked by the original grantee institution, as they want their incoming recruits to bring awards as well.

If you are anticipating an NoA and know you are changing jobs, you may be able to delay the NoA such that it can be made directly to your new institution (pending appropriate paperwork). You should discuss the possibility of delaying the Notice with your PO as part of your preparation to have the award transferred. You should not be afraid that merely telling your PO about a new job will endanger your award; however, if the new institution is not eligible or appropriate for the research proposed, this is a different situation, as noted earlier.

If your Notice cannot be delayed (often the case for awards at the end of the fiscal year) and arrives in the midst of your move, you can ask your original institution not to activate the award (i.e., not to draw on any of the funds) until it can be transferred. This is a discussion you would need to have with your department and the office of sponsored programs or research at your current (awarded) institution rather than anyone at the NIH.

Carryover

Given the uncertainties of funding, many PIs are conservative in spending their award so as to cover their laboratory beyond the approved award period. You should review your NoA for any restrictions on carryover (varies by mechanism and can include special IC-specific limitations). Generally, you can carry over funds from year to year (policy at the time of this writing available here, http://grants.nih.gov/grants/policy/nihgps_2012/nihgps_ch8.htm#_Toc271264925), though your terms of award will indicate the circumstances in which you may need to provide an explanation for the unobligated balance (usually triggered if the unobligated balance exceeds 25% of the annual budget) and scientific justification for use of the funds in the subsequent year (plus the budget information itself).

At the conclusion of your final award year, you will notify your IC that you are exercising your authority to extend existing funds beyond the project period, known as a No-Cost Extension (NCE), which does not require prior approval unless the terms of your award indicate otherwise (http://grants.nih.gov/grants/policy/nihgps_2012/nihgps_ch8.htm#_Toc271264927). You can do this while your competing renewal (Type 2) application is pending or even if you did not submit a competing renewal (particularly for those mechanisms that cannot be renewed). If you still have funds at the end of your first year of NCE, you will need advance permission from your PO to carry any remaining monies into a second year.

Keeping the Money Coming: NIH Public Access Policy

Your noncompeting renewal awards (Type 5) are issued after you submit your annual Research Performance Progress Report (http://grants.nih.gov/grants/rppr/index.htm) via eRA Commons, for awards issued under the Streamlined Noncompeting Award Process (SNAP), fellowships, and eventually all non-SNAP awards (explained in the current NIH Grants Policy Statement, http://grants1.nih.gov/grants/policy/policy.htm). One component that could determine whether you continue to receive funding is your compliance with the NIH Public Access Policy (http://publicaccess.nih.gov/index.htm). You must submit to PubMed Central (http://www.ncbi.nlm.nih.gov/pmc/), upon acceptance for publication, all final peer-reviewed journal manuscripts reporting research funded by an NIH grant award—and you in fact should want to link your publications to your NIH awards. Doing so helps you with your competing renewal and helps your PO in justifying his or her portfolio—not to mention your IC in justifying their budget request to Congress.

You will use My NCBI (http://www.ncbi.nlm.nih.gov/books/NBK3842/) to generate a PDF report of these publications, including their PubMed Central (PMCID) or, while final deposition is pending, NIH Manuscript Submission ID (NIHMSID) numbers for inclusion in your progress report. When selecting target journals for your manuscripts, be sure to pay attention to whether they will deposit your manuscript in PubMed Central for you and whether there are any copyright restrictions that you must address at the time you submit your manuscript.

One final comment with regard to publications that result from your NIH funding: be sure to cite your award(s) by the complete grant number (e.g., R01CA010101) rather than by title (BPSI for Studying DNA Repair), partial number (e.g., CA010101), or general reference (e.g., NCI R01). When POs search PubMed for publications linked to awards in their portfolio, they do so by grant number rather than by PI or other terms, and you want to be sure your publications are found.

Contacts and Resources at Institutes and Centers

HERE WE PRESENT a common dataset for all the Institutes followed by the Centers (ICs; listed alphabetically by name, not abbreviation) that will help you navigate each IC Web site more efficiently and find the information you need to start the conversation with your Program Officer (PO) or other program staff. Please remember that IC Web sites are continually updated and that you may need to search for information that has moved. You can also check the Writedit blog, Medical Writing, Editing & Grantsmanship (http://writedit. wordpress.com), for updated links and information.

National Cancer Institute (NCI)
http://cancer.gov

National Cancer Advisory Board
http://deainfo.nci.nih.gov/advisory/ncab/ncab.htm

Review Groups
http://deainfo.nci.nih.gov/advisory/irg/irg.htm
http://deainfo.nci.nih.gov/advisory/sep/sep.htm

Cleared Concepts
http://deainfo.nci.nih.gov/concepts/concepts.htm

Funding Announcements
http://cancer.gov/researchandfunding/funding/announcements

Funding Units and Scientific Contacts
http://www.cancer.gov/researchandfunding/contacts
- *Cancer Biology*: https://dcb.nci.nih.gov/About/Pages/StaffByResearchExpertise.aspx
- *Cancer Control and Population Sciences*: http://cancercontrol.cancer.gov/od/meet_staff.html
- *Cancer Prevention*: http://prevention.cancer.gov/about/staff/dcp
- *Cancer Treatment and Diagnosis*: http://dctd.cancer.gov/About/default.htm

Grants Management Staff
http://www3.cancer.gov/admin/gab/phones.htm

Training/Career Development
http://cancer.gov/researchandfunding/trainingopportunities

Small Business Resources (SBIR/STTR)
http://sbir.cancer.gov/

National Eye Institute (NEI)
http://www.nei.nih.gov

National Advisory Eye Council
http://nei.nih.gov/about/naec/index.asp

Review Groups
http://era.nih.gov/roster/Proster1.cfm?ABBR=ZEY1&CID=100566

Cleared Concepts
http://www.nei.nih.gov/about/naec/mom.asp (click on latest Council minutes)

Funding Announcements
http://www.nei.nih.gov/funding/app.asp

Funding Units and Scientific Contacts
http://nei.nih.gov/funding/extram.asp
http://nei.nih.gov/funding/nprp.asp

Grants Management Staff
http://nei.nih.gov/funding/extram.asp (scroll down to Grants Management Staff)

Training/Career Development
http://grants1.nih.gov/training/extramural.htm

Small Business Resources (SBIR/STTR)
http://grants.nih.gov/grants/funding/sbir.htm

National Heart, Lung and Blood Institute (NHLBI)
http://www.nhlbi.nih.gov/

National Heart, Lung and Blood Advisory Council
http://www.nhlbi.nih.gov/meetings/nhlbac/index.htm

Review Groups
http://www.nhlbi.nih.gov/about/advisory.htm#peer

Cleared Concepts
http://www.nhlbi.nih.gov/meetings/nhlbac/ (click on latest Council
   minutes)

Funding Announcements
http://www.nhlbi.nih.gov/funding/inits/index.htm
http://www.nhlbi.nih.gov/resources/listserv/index.htm (LISTSERV)

Funding Units and Scientific Contacts
http://www.nhlbi.nih.gov/about/staff-expertise.htm
- *Blood Diseases and Resources*: http://www.nhlbi.nih.gov/about/
   dbdr/index.htm
- *Cardiovascular Sciences*: http://www.nhlbi.nih.gov/about/dcvd/
   index.htm
- *Lung Diseases*: http://www.nhlbi.nih.gov/about/dld/index.htm

Grants Management Staff
http://www.nhlbi.nih.gov/about/staff-expertise.htm (scroll down to
   Office of Grants Management)
http://www.nhlbi.nih.gov/about/dera/index.htm

Training/Career Development
http://www.nhlbi.nih.gov/training/index.htm

Small Business Resources (SBIR/STTR)
http://www.nhlbi.nih.gov/funding/sbir/index.htm

National Human Genome Research Institute (NHGRI)
http://www.genome.gov

National Advisory Council for Human Genome Research
http://www.genome.gov/10000905

Review Groups

http://www.genome.gov/10000917

Cleared Concepts

http://www.genome.gov/10000905 (click on most recent Council
  meeting)

Funding Announcements

http://www.genome.gov/10000884#al-3
http://www.genome.gov/10000259 (LISTSERV)

Funding Units and Scientific Contacts

http://www.genome.gov/27550076

- *Genomic Medicine*: http://www.genome.gov/27550610
- *Genomic Sciences*: http://www.genome.gov/27550609
- *Genomics and Society*: http://www.genome.gov/27550080

Grants Management Staff

http://www.genome.gov/10001181

Training/Career Development

http://www.genome.gov/10000950

Small Business Resources (SBIR/STTR)

http://grants.nih.gov/grants/funding/sbir.htm

National Institute on Aging (NIA)

http://www.nia.nih.gov

National Advisory Council on Aging

http://www.nia.nih.gov/about/naca

Review Groups

http://www.nia.nih.gov/research/dea-scientific-review

Cleared Concepts

http://www.nia.nih.gov/about/naca (click on most recent Council
  meeting)

Funding Announcements

http://www.nia.nih.gov/research/funding

Funding Units and Scientific Contacts

- *Aging Biology*: http://www.nia.nih.gov/research/dab
- *Behavioral and Social Research*: http://www.nia.nih.gov/
  research/dbsr

- *Geriatrics and Clinical Gerontology*: http://www.nia.nih.gov/research/dgcg
- *Neuroscience*: http://www.nia.nih.gov/research/dn

Grants Management Staff
http://www.nia.nih.gov/about/staff?title=&field_nihsac3_tid=3147&field_location_tid=All

Training/Career Development
http://www.nia.nih.gov/research/dea/research-training-and-career-award-support

Small Business Resources (SBIR/STTR)
http://www.nia.nih.gov/research/dea/small-business-innovation-research-sbir

National Institute of Alcohol Abuse and Alcoholism (NIAAA)
http://www.niaaa.nih.gov

National Advisory Council on Alcohol Abuse and Alcoholism
http://www.niaaa.nih.gov/about-niaaa/our-work/advisory-council

Review Groups
http://www.niaaa.nih.gov/grant-funding/application-process/niaaa-scientific-review-group-rosters

Cleared Concepts
http://www.niaaa.nih.gov/about-niaaa/our-work/advisory-council/agenda-minutes/advisory-council-meeting-minutes (click on most recent Council minutes)

Funding Announcements
http://www.niaaa.nih.gov/grant-funding/funding-opportunities

Funding Units and Scientific Contacts
http://www.niaaa.nih.gov/grant-funding/application-process (scroll down to Contacts for Additional Questions)

Training/Career Development
http://www.niaaa.nih.gov/ResearchInformation/ExtramuralResearch

Small Business Resources (SBIR/STTR)
http://grants.nih.gov/grants/funding/sbir.htm

National Institute of Allergy and Infectious Diseases (NIAID)
http://www.niaid.nih.gov

National Advisory Allergy and Infectious Diseases Council
http://www.niaid.nih.gov/researchfunding/council/Pages/default.aspx

Review Groups
http://era.nih.gov/roster/roster.cfm?cid=100236&cn=acquired%20
immunodeficiency%20syndrome%20research%20review%20 committee
http://era.nih.gov/roster/roster.cfm?cid=100231&cn=allergy%2c%20
immunology%2c%20and%20transplantation%20research%20
committee
http://era.nih.gov/roster/roster.cfm?cid=100235&cn=microbiology%20
and%20infectious%20diseases%20research%20committee
http://era.nih.gov/roster/roster.cfm?cid=103124&cn=microbiology%20
and%20infectious%20diseases%20b%20subcommittee

Cleared Concepts
http://www.niaid.nih.gov/researchfunding/council/concepts/Pages/
default.aspx

Funding Announcements
http://www.niaid.nih.gov/researchfunding/ann/Pages/opps.aspx
http://www.niaid.nih.gov/researchfunding/newsletter/pages/subscribe.
aspx (LISTSERV)

Funding Units and Scientific Contacts
http://www.niaid.nih.gov/researchfunding/grant/strategy/Pages/
contacttips.aspx
http://www.niaid.nih.gov/researchfunding/grant/checklists/Pages/
checkpo.aspx

- *AIDS*: http://www.niaid.nih.gov/about/findingpeople/pages/
daids.aspx
- *Allergy, Immunology, and Transplantation*: http://www.niaid.
nih.gov/about/findingpeople/pages/dait.aspx
- *Microbiology and Infectious Diseases*: http://www.niaid.nih.gov/
about/findingpeople/Pages/dmid_staff.aspx

Grants Management Staff
http://www.niaid.nih.gov/about/organization/dea/Pages/gmp.aspx

Training/Career Development
http://www.niaid.nih.gov/researchfunding/traincareer/Pages/default.aspx

Small Business Resources (SBIR/STTR)
http://www.niaid.nih.gov/researchfunding/sb/Pages/default.aspx

National Institute of Arthritis and Musculoskeletal and Skin Diseases (NIAMS)
http://www.niams.nih.gov/

National Arthritis and Musculoskeletal and Skin Diseases Advisory Council
http://www.niams.nih.gov/About_Us/Committees/council_roster.asp

Review Groups
http://era.nih.gov/roster/proster.cfm?CID=100265
http://era.nih.gov/roster/proster.cfm?CID=104156
http://www.niams.nih.gov/Funding/Funding_Process/Rosters/default.asp

Cleared Concepts
http://www.niams.nih.gov/News_and_Events/Advisory_Council_Minutes/ (click on most recent Council minutes)

Funding Announcements
http://www.niams.nih.gov/Funding/Funding_Opportunities/default.asp

Funding Units and Scientific Contacts
http://www.niams.nih.gov/Funding/Funding_Opportunities/Supported_Scientific_Areas/default.asp
- *Skin and Rheumatic Diseases*: http://www.niams.nih.gov/Funding/Funding_Opportunities/Supported_Scientific_Areas/Skin_Rheumatic_Diseases/default.asp
- *Musculoskeletal Diseases*: http://www.niams.nih.gov/Funding/Funding_Opportunities/Supported_Scientific_Areas/Musculoskeletal_Diseases/default.asp

Grants Management Staff
http://www.niams.nih.gov/Funding/Funding_Process/Portfolio_Assignment.asp

Training/Career Development
http://www.niams.nih.gov/Funding/Funding_Opportunities/activity_codes.asp#1&Fellowship Programs (F) (scroll down to next section for Career Development/K awards)

Small Business Resources (SBIR/STTR)

http://grants.nih.gov/grants/funding/sbir.htm

National Institute of Biomedical Imaging and Bioengineering (NIBIB)
http://www.nibib.nih.gov/

National Advisory Council for Biomedical Imaging and Bioengineering
http://www.nibib.nih.gov/About/AdvisoryCouncil

Review Groups
http://era.nih.gov/roster/Proster1.cfm?ABBR=ZEB1&CID=102436

Cleared Concepts
http://www.nibib.nih.gov/About/AdvisoryCouncil/ (click on most recent Council minutes)

Funding Announcements
http://www.nibib.nih.gov/funding/funding-opportunities
https://list.nih.gov/cgi-bin/wa.exe?SUBED1=NIBIB_LISTSERV&A=1

Funding Units and Scientific Contacts
http://www.nibib.nih.gov/Research/ProgramAreas
http://www.nibib.nih.gov/about-nibib/staff

Grants Management Staff
http://www.nibib.nih.gov/about-nibib/staff

Training/Career Development
http://www.nibib.nih.gov/training-careers

Small Business Resources (SBIR/STTR)
http://www.nibib.nih.gov/funding/funding-policies/small-business-innovation-research-and-small-business-technology-transfer

Eunice Kennedy Shriver National Institute of Child Health and Human Development (NICHD)
http://www.nichd.nih.gov/

National Advisory Child Health and Human Development Council
http://www.nichd.nih.gov/about/advisory/nachhd/Pages/index.aspx

Review Groups
http://www.nichd.nih.gov/grants-funding/peer-review/Pages/default.aspx

Cleared Concepts

http://www.nichd.nih.gov/grants-funding/opportunities-mechanisms/
proposed-opportunities/Pages/default.aspx

Funding Announcements

http://www.nichd.nih.gov/grants-funding/opportunities-mechanisms/
Pages/default.aspx

Funding Units and Scientific Contacts

http://www.nichd.nih.gov/about/org/der/branches/Pages/index.aspx

Grants Management Staff

http://www.nichd.nih.gov/about/org/od/oam/index.cfm

Training/Career Development

http://www.nichd.nih.gov/training/Pages/default.aspx

Small Business Resources (SBIR/STTR)

http://www.nichd.nih.gov/grants-funding/opportunities-mechanisms/
mechanisms-types/small-business-mechanisms/Pages/default.aspx

**National Institute of Deafness and Other Communication Disorders
(NIDCD)**

http://www.nidcd.nih.gov/

**National Deafness and Other Communication Disorders Advisory
Council**

http://www.nidcd.nih.gov/about/groups/ndcdac/Pages/default.aspx

Review Groups

http://www.nidcd.nih.gov/about/groups/cdrc/Pages/defaultpage.aspx
http://www.nidcd.nih.gov/about/groups/sep/Pages/defaultpage.aspx

Cleared Concepts

http://www.nidcd.nih.gov/about/groups/ndcdac/pages/minutes.aspx
(click on most recent Council minutes)

Funding Announcements

http://www.nidcd.nih.gov/funding/Pages/Default.aspx

Funding Units and Scientific Contacts

http://www.nidcd.nih.gov/funding/apply/pages/staff.aspx
- *Hearing*: http://www.nidcd.nih.gov/funding/programs/pages/
descripth.aspx

- *Balance*: http://www.nidcd.nih.gov/funding/programs/pages/descriptb.aspx
  http://www.nidcd.nih.gov/funding/programs/pages/descriptst.aspx
- *Voice, Speech, and Language*: http://www.nidcd.nih.gov/funding/programs/pages/descriptvsl.aspx

Grants Management Staff
http://www.nidcd.nih.gov/about/staff/pages/der.aspx

Training/Career Development
http://www.nidcd.nih.gov/research/training/Pages/Default.aspx

Small Business Resources (SBIR/STTR)
http://www.nidcd.nih.gov/funding/types/pages/smallbusiness.aspx

National Institute of Dental and Craniofacial Research (NIDCR)
http://www.nidcr.nih.gov/

National Advisory Dental and Craniofacial Research Council
http://www.nidcr.nih.gov/AboutUs/Councils/NADCRC/

Review Groups
http://www.nidcr.nih.gov/AboutUs/Councils/SGR/
http://www.nidcr.nih.gov/AboutUs/Councils/SEP/

Cleared Concepts
http://www.nidcr.nih.gov/GrantsAndFunding/See_Funding_Opportunities_Sorted_By/ConceptClearance/CurrentCC/default.htm

Funding Announcements
http://www.nidcr.nih.gov/GrantsAndFunding/FundingOpportunityAnnouncements/ByTopic.htm

Funding Units and Scientific Contacts
http://www.nidcr.nih.gov/Research/DER/DEROverview
http://www.nidcr.nih.gov/Research/DER/ContactRA.htm
- *Behavioral and Social Sciences*: http://www.nidcr.nih.gov/Research/DER/BSSRB
- *Clinical Research*: http://www.nidcr.nih.gov/Research/DER/ClinicalResearch/
- *Integrative Biology and Infectious Diseases*: http://www.nidcr.nih.gov/Research/DER/IntegrativeBiologyAndInfectious Diseases/

- *Translational Genomics*: http://www.nidcr.nih.gov/Research/
  DER/TGRB

Grants Management Staff
http://www.nidcr.nih.gov/AboutUs/StaffDirectoryandOrganization/
  OrganizationalCharts/DivisionofExtramuralActivities/ByBranch.
  htm#GrantsManagementBranch

Training/Career Development
http://www.nidcr.nih.gov/careersandtraining/

Small Business Resources (SBIR/STTR)
http://www.nidcr.nih.gov/AtoZ/LetterS/SBIRSTTR/

National Institute of Diabetes and Digestive and Kidney Disease (NIDDK)
http://www.niddk.nih.gov/

National Diabetes and Digestive and Kidney Disease Advisory Council
http://www2.niddk.nih.gov/AboutNIDDK/ResearchAndPlanning/
  AdvisoryCouncil/

Review Groups
http://www2.niddk.nih.gov/Funding/Grants/GrantReview/
  ReviewRosters.htm
http://www2.niddk.nih.gov/Funding/Grants/GrantReview/Review_
  Staff.htm

Cleared Concepts
http://www2.niddk.nih.gov/AboutNIDDK/ResearchAndPlanning/
  AdvisoryCouncil/Meetings/Default (click on most recent Council
  minutes)

Funding Announcements
http://www2.niddk.nih.gov/Funding/FundingOpportunities/

Funding Units and Scientific Contacts
http://www2.niddk.nih.gov/Research/ScientificAreas/
- *Diabetes, Endocrinology, and Metabolic Diseases*: http://www2.
  niddk.nih.gov/AboutNIDDK/NIDDKStaff/Biosketches/DEM/
- *Digestive Diseases and Nutrition*: http://www2.niddk.nih.gov/
  AboutNIDDK/NIDDKStaff/Biosketches/DDN/

- *Kidney, Urologic, and Hematologic Diseases*: http://www2. niddk.nih.gov/AboutNIDDK/NIDDKStaff/Biosketches/ DKUH/

Grants Management Staff
http://www2.niddk.nih.gov/Funding/Grants/GrantsManagement.htm

Training/Career Development
http://www2.niddk.nih.gov/Funding/TrainingCareerDev/

Small Business Resources (SBIR/STTR)
http://www2.niddk.nih.gov/Funding/SmallBusiness/

National Institute on Drug Abuse (NIDA)
http://www.drugabuse.gov/

National Advisory Council on Drug Abuse
http://www.drugabuse.gov/about-nida/advisory-boards-groups/ national-advisory-council-drug-abuse-nacda

Review Groups
http://www.drugabuse.gov/about-nida/advisory-boards-review-groups/ scientific-review-groupcommittee-structure

Cleared Concepts
http://www.drugabuse.gov/about-nida/advisory-boards-groups/ national-advisory-council-drug-abuse-nacda/council-meeting-min-utes (click on most recent Council minutes)

Funding Announcements
http://www.drugabuse.gov/funding/funding-opportunities

Funding Units and Scientific Contacts
http://www.drugabuse.gov/about-nida/organization
- *Basic Neuroscience and Behavioral Research*: http://www. drugabuse.gov/about-nida/organization/divisions/division-basic-neuroscience-behavioral-research-dbnbr
- *Clinical Neuroscience and Behavioral Research*: http://www.dru-gabuse.gov/about-nida/organization/divisions/division-clinical-neuroscience-behavioral-research-dcnbr
- *Epidemiology, Services and Prevention Research*: http://www. drugabuse.gov/about-nida/organization/divisions/division-epidemiology-services-prevention-research-despr

- *Pharmacotherapies and Medical Consequences of Drug Abuse*: http://www.drugabuse.gov/about-nida/organization/ divisions/division-pharmacotherapies-medical-consequences-drug-abuse-dpmcda
- *Clinical Trials Network*: http://www.drugabuse.gov/about-nida/ organization/cctn

Grants Management Staff
http://www.drugabuse.gov/about-nida/organization/offices/office-management-om

Training/Career Development
http://www.drugabuse.gov/funding/research-training

Small Business Resources (SBIR/STTR)
http://www.drugabuse.gov/funding/funding-opportunities/small-business-funding

National Institute of Environmental Health Sciences (NIEHS)
http://www.niehs.nih.gov

National Advisory Environmental Health Sciences Council
http://www.niehs.nih.gov/about/boards/naehsc/index.cfm

Review Groups
http://www.niehs.nih.gov/research/supported/dert/srb/index.cfm

Cleared Concepts
http://www.niehs.nih.gov/about/boards/naehsc/ (click on most recent Council minutes)

Funding Announcements
http://www.niehs.nih.gov/funding/index.cfm

Funding Units and Scientific Contacts
http://www.niehs.nih.gov/funding/grants/contacts/index.cfm
- *Cellular, Organs, and Systems Pathobiology*: http://www.niehs. nih.gov/research/supported/dert/cospb/index.cfm
- *Risk and Integrated Sciences*: http://www.niehs.nih.gov/research/ supported/dert/cris/index.cfm
- *Susceptibility and Population Health*: http://www.niehs.nih.gov/ research/supported/dert/sphb/index.cfm

Grants Management Staff
http://www.niehs.nih.gov/research/supported/dert/gmb/index.cfm

Training/Career Development
http://www.niehs.nih.gov/careers/research/index.cfm

Small Business Resources (SBIR/STTR)
http://www.niehs.nih.gov/funding/grants/mechanisms/sbir/index.cfm

National Institute of General Medical Sciences Sciences (NIGMS)
http://www.nigms.nih.gov

National Advisory General Medical Sciences Council
http://www.nigms.nih.gov/About/Council/

Review Groups
http://www.csr.nih.gov/Roster_proto/cmtelist2.asp?Title=National
+Institute+of+General+Medic http://era.nih.gov/roster/Proster1.
cfm?ABBR=ZGM1&CID=100647 al+Sciences+Initial+Review+
Group&ABBR=BRT

http://public.nigms.nih.gov/StaffContacts/index.cfm?event=search_
results&sort_by=&last_name=&first_name=&component_id=10

Cleared Concepts
http://www.nigms.nih.gov/About/Council/Minutes/ (click on most
recent Council minutes)

Funding Announcements
http://search.nigms.nih.gov/funding/funding.asp?tab=All

Funding Units and Scientific Contacts
http://www.nigms.nih.gov/About/ContactByArea.htm
- *Biomedical Technology, Bioinformatics, and Computational
Biology*: http://www.nigms.nih.gov/About/Overview/bbcb.htm
- *Cell Biology and Biophysics*: http://www.nigms.nih.gov/About/
Overview/CBB.htm
- *Genetics and Developmental Biology*: http://www.nigms.nih.
gov/About/Overview/gdb.htm
- *Pharmacology, Physiology, and Biological Chemistry*: http://
www.nigms.nih.gov/About/Overview/ppbc.htm

Grants Management Staff
http://public.nigms.nih.gov/StaffContacts/ and select Grants
Administration Branch

Training/Career Development

http://www.nigms.nih.gov/About/Overview/twd.htm

Small Business Resources (SBIR/STTR)

http://www.nigms.nih.gov/Research/Mechanisms/SBIR.htm

http://www.nigms.nih.gov/Research/Mechanisms/STTR.htm

National Institute of Mental Health (NIMH)

http://www.nihm.nih.gov

National Advisory Mental Health Council

http://www.nimh.nih.gov/about/advisory-boards-and-groups/namhc/
index.shtml

Review Groups

http://www.nimh.nih.gov/research-funding/grants/peer-review-
committees.shtml

Cleared Concepts

http://www.nimh.nih.gov/about/advisory-boards-and-groups/namhc/
namhc-concept-clearances.shtml

Funding Announcements

http://www.nimh.nih.gov/research-funding/grants/opportunities-
announcements/index.shtml

Funding Units and Scientific Contacts

http://www.nimh.nih.gov/about/organization/extramural-programs-
and-contacts-listed-by-division.shtml

- *Neuroscience and Basic Behavioral Science*: http://www.nimh.
  nih.gov/about/organization/dnbbs/index.shtml
- *Adult Translational Research and Treatment Development*: http://www.nimh.nih.gov/about/organization/datr/index.
  shtml
- *Developmental Translational Research*: http://www.nimh.nih.
  gov/about/organization/ddtr/index.shtml
- *AIDS Research*: http://www.nimh.nih.gov/about/organization/
  dar/index.shtml
- *Services and Intervention Research*: http://www.nimh.nih.gov/
  about/organization/dsir/index.shtml

Grants Management Staff

http://www.nimh.nih.gov/about/staff-directories/headquarters-hq-and-
extramural-staff-organizational-locator.shtml

Training/Career Development
http://www.nimh.nih.gov/research-funding/training/index.shtml

Small Business Resources (SBIR/STTR)
http://www.nimh.nih.gov/research-funding/small-business/index.shtml

National Institute of Minority Health and Health Disparities (NIMHD)
http://www.nimhd.nih.gov

National Advisory Council on Minority Health and Health Disparities
http://www.nimhd.nih.gov/about_ncmhd/advise.asp

Funding Units and Scientific Contacts
http://www.nimhd.nih.gov/about_ncmhd/contact.asp

Grants Management Staff

Training/Career Development
http://grants1.nih.gov/training/extramural.htm

Small Business Resources (SBIR/STTR)
http://www.nimhd.nih.gov/our_programs/smallBusinessresearch
    Technology.asp

National Institute of Neurological Disorders and Stroke (NINDS)
http://www.ninds.nih.gov

National Advisory Neurological Disorders and Stroke Council
    http://www.ninds.nih.gov/find_people/nands/index.htm

Review Groups
http://www.ninds.nih.gov/funding/review_committees/index.htm

Cleared Concepts
http://www.ninds.nih.gov/find_people/nands/index.htm#Minutes
    (click on most recent Council minutes)

Funding Announcements
http://www.ninds.nih.gov/funding/funding_announcements/funding_
    opps.htm

Funding Units and Scientific Contacts
http://www.ninds.nih.gov/find_people/ninds/contact_people.htm
http://www.ninds.nih.gov/funding/pd_interests.pdf
  • *Channels, Synapses, and Neural Circuits*: http://www.ninds.nih.
    gov/funding/areas/channels_synapses_and_circuits/index.htm

- *Neural Environment*: http://www.ninds.nih.gov/funding/areas/ neural_environment/index.htm
- *Neurodegeneration*: http://www.ninds.nih.gov/funding/areas/ neurodegeneration/index.htm
- *Neurogenetics*: http://www.ninds.nih.gov/funding/areas/ neurogenetics/index.htm
- *Repair and Plasticity*: http://www.ninds.nih.gov/funding/areas/ repair_and_plasticity/index.htm
- *Systems and Cognitive Neuroscience*: http://www.ninds.nih.gov/ funding/areas/systems_and_cognitive_neuroscience/index.htm
- *Clinical Research*: http://www.ninds.nih.gov/research/clinical_ research/index.htm
- *International Activities*: http://www.ninds.nih.gov/funding/ areas/office_of_international_activities/index.htm

Grants Management Staff
http://www.ninds.nih.gov/funding/grants_management_branch/index. htm

Training/Career Development
http://www.ninds.nih.gov/funding/areas/training_and_career_ development/index.htm

Small Business Resources (SBIR/STTR)
http://www.ninds.nih.gov/funding/small-business/index.htm

National Institute of Nursing Research (NINR)

National Advisory Council for Nursing Research
http://www.ninr.nih.gov/AboutNINR/NACNR/

Review Groups
http://www.ninr.nih.gov/ResearchAndFunding/DEA/OR/

Cleared Concepts
http://www.ninr.nih.gov/aboutninr/nacnr (click on most recent Council minutes)

Funding Announcements
http://www.ninr.nih.gov/ResearchAndFunding/DEA/OEP/ FundingOpportunities/default.htm

Funding Units and Scientific Contacts

http://www.ninr.nih.gov/ResearchAndFunding/DEA/OEP/
   AreasofscienceFile.htm (cross-cutting areas and special mechanisms
   at the bottom)

- *Neuroscience, Genetics, and Symptom Management*: http://
  www.ninr.nih.gov/ResearchAndFunding/DEA/OEP/
  AreasofscienceFile.htm#NEURO
- *Child and Family Health, and Health Disparities*: http://
  www.ninr.nih.gov/ResearchAndFunding/DEA/OEP/
  AreasofscienceFile.htm#CHILD
- *Immunology, Infectious Disease, and Chronic Disorders*: http://
  www.ninr.nih.gov/ResearchAndFunding/DEA/OEP/
  AreasofscienceFile.htm#IMMUNE
- *Acute and Long-Term Care, End of Life, and Training*: http://
  www.ninr.nih.gov/ResearchAndFunding/DEA/OEP/
  AreasofscienceFile.htm#ACUTE

Grants Management Staff

http://www.ninr.nih.gov/ResearchAndFunding/DEA/OGM/

Training/Career Development

http://www.ninr.nih.gov/Training/TrainingOpportunitiesExtramural/

Small Business Resources (SBIR/STTR)

http://grants.nih.gov/grants/funding/sbir.htm

National Library of Medicine (NLM)

http://www.nlm.nih.gov

NLM Board of Regents

http://www.nlm.nih.gov/od/bor/bor.html

Review Groups

http://www.nlm.nih.gov/ep/Staff.html (scroll down to Scientific Review
   Office, links to SRG rosters at bottom of page)

Cleared Concepts

http://www.nlm.nih.gov/od/bor/bor.html (click on most recent Board
   of Regents minutes)

Funding Announcements

http://www.nlm.nih.gov/ep/Grants.html

Funding Units and Scientific Contacts

http://www.nlm.nih.gov/ep/Staff.html (scroll down to Program Office)

Grants Management Staff

http://www.nlm.nih.gov/ep/Staff.html (scroll down to Grants
  Management Office)

NLM POs schedule one-on-one meetings to discuss proposed project
  ideas with a PI

Training/Career Development

http://www.nlm.nih.gov/ep/Grants.html#career

Small Business Resources (SBIR/STTR)

http://www.nlm.nih.gov/ep/Grants.html#small

**John E. Fogarty International Center for the Advanced Study in the
  Health Sciences (FIC)**

http://www.fic.nih.gov/

Fogarty Advisory Board

http://www.fic.nih.gov/About/Advisory/Pages/default.aspx

Review Groups

None within the Center

Cleared Concepts

http://www.fic.nih.gov/About/Advisory/Pages/default.aspx (click on
  most recent Board minutes)

Funding Announcements

http://www.fic.nih.gov/Funding/Pages/default.aspx
https://public.govdelivery.com/accounts/USNIHFIC/subscriber/new
  (LISTSERV)

Funding Units and Scientific Contacts

http://www.fic.nih.gov/About/Staff/Pages/Training-Research.aspx
http://www.fic.nih.gov/About/Staff/Pages/staff-directory-subject-area.
  aspx

Training/Career Development

http://www.fic.nih.gov/Programs/Pages/default.aspx (see Career
  Development Opportunities)

Grants Management Staff

http://www.fic.nih.gov/About/Staff/Pages/staff-directory.aspx (scroll to
  Grants Management)

Small Business Resources (SBIR/STTR)

http://grants.nih.gov/grants/funding/sbir.htm

National Center for Advancing Translational Sciences (NCATS)
http://www.ncats.nih.gov

NCATS Advisory Council
http://www.ncats.nih.gov/about/ncats-council/council.html

Review Groups
http://era.nih.gov/roster/Proster1.cfm?ABBR=ZTR1&CID=104162

Cleared Concepts
http://www.ncats.nih.gov/about/ncats-council/council.html (click on
   most recent Council minutes)

Funding Announcements
http://www.ncats.nih.gov/funding-and-notices/funding.html
http://nih.us5.list-manage.com/subscribe?u=e06bd55ccbb41f1a362306d
   ff&id=fc1085e209 (LISTSERV)

Funding Units and Scientific Contacts
http://www.ncats.nih.gov/about/contact-us/contact-us.html
http://www.ncats.nih.gov/about/org/divs-offices/divisions-offices.html

Grants Management Staff
http://www.ncats.nih.gov/about/contact-us/contact-us.html

Training/Career Development
http://grants1.nih.gov/training/extramural.htm

Small Business Resources (SBIR/STTR)
http://www.ncats.nih.gov/funding-and-notices/small-business/small-
   business.html

**National Center for Complementary and Alternative Medicine
   (NCCAM)**
http://nccam.nih.gov

**National Advisory Council for Complementary and Alternative
   Medicine**
http://nccam.nih.gov/about/naccam

Review Groups
http://era.nih.gov/roster/Proster1.cfm?ABBR=ZAT1&CID=101760
http://nccam.nih.gov/about/offices/osr

Cleared Concepts
http://nccam.nih.gov/grants/concepts

Funding Announcements
http://nccam.nih.gov/grants/funding

Funding Units and Scientific Contacts
http://nccam.nih.gov/grants/contact

Grants Management Staff
http://nccam.nih.gov/about/offices/ogm

Training/Career Development
http://www.nccam.nih.gov/training

Small Business Resources (SBIR/STTR)
http://www.nccam.nih.gov/grants/types/sbirsttr

Index